General Orthopedics

Editor

KARA-ANN VALENTINE

PHYSICIAN ASSISTANT CLINICS

www.physicianassistant.theclinics.com

Consulting Editors
KIM ZUBER
JANE S. DAVIS

January 2024 • Volume 9 • Number 1

ELSEVIER

1600 John F. Kennedy Boulevard • Suite 1800 • Philadelphia, Pennsylvania, 19103-2899

http://www.theclinics.com

PHYSICIAN ASSISTANT CLINICS Volume 9, Number 1
January 2024 ISSN 2405-7991, ISBN-13: 978-0-443-18384-3

Editor: Taylor Hayes
Developmental Editor: Saswoti Nath

Physician Assistant Clinics (ISSN: 2405–7991) is published quarterly by Elsevier Inc., 360 Park Avenue South, New York, NY 10010-1710. Months of issue are January, April, July, and October. Periodicals postage paid at New York, NY and additional mailing offices. Subscription prices are $155.00 per year (US individuals), $100.00 (US students), $150.00 (Canadian individuals), $100.00 (Canadian students), $150.00 (international individuals), and $100.00 (international students). For institutional access pricing please contact Customer Service via the contact information below. Foreign air speed delivery is included in all *Clinics* subscription prices. All prices are subject to change without notice. POSTMASTER: Send address changes to *Physician Assistant Clinics*, Elsevier Periodicals Customer Service, 11830 Westline Industrial Drive, St. Louis, MO 63146. Customer Service Health Sciences Division, Subscription Customer Service, 3251 Riverport Lane, Maryland Heights, MO 63043. **Customer Service: 1-800-654-2452 (U.S. and Canada); 314-447-8871 (outside U.S. and Canada). Fax: 314-447-8029. E-mail: journalscustomerservice-usa@elsevier.com (for print support); journalsonlinesupport-usa@elsevier.com (for online support).**

Reprints. For copies of 100 or more, of articles in this publication, please contact the Commercial Reprints Department, Elsevier Inc., 360 Park Avenue South, New York, NY 10010-1710. Tel. 212-633-3874; Fax: 212-633-3820; E-mail: reprints@elsevier.com.

Physician Assistant Clinics is covered in *EMBASE/Excerpta Medica and ESCI*.

PROGRAM OBJECTIVE

The goal of the *Physician Assistant Clinics* is to keep practicing physician assistants up to date with current clinical practice by providing timely articles reviewing the state of the art in patient care.

TARGET AUDIENCE

Physician Assistants and other healthcare professionals

LEARNING OBJECTIVES

Upon completion of this activity, participants will be able to:

1. Review the incidences and risk factors associated with musculoskeletal injuries.
2. Discuss the essential role orthopedics plays in the everyday health and mobility of people all over the world.
3. Recognize the importance of collaboration with various other subspecialties in evaluating and managing musculoskeletal injuries and conditions.

ACCREDITATION

The Elsevier Office of Continuing Medical Education (EOCME) is accredited by the Accreditation Council for Continuing Medical Education (ACCME) to provide continuing medical education for physicians.

The EOCME designates this journal-based CME activity for a maximum of 13 *AMA PRA Category 1 Credit*(s)™. Physicians should claim only the credit commensurate with the extent of their participation in the activity.

All other health care professionals requesting continuing education credit for this enduring material will be issued a certificate of participation.

DISCLOSURE OF CONFLICTS OF INTEREST

The EOCME assesses conflict of interest with its instructors, faculty, planners, and other individuals who are in a position to control the content of CME activities. All relevant conflicts of interest that are identified are thoroughly vetted by EOCME for fair balance, scientific objectivity, and patient care recommendations. EOCME is committed to providing its learners with CME activities that promote improvements or quality in healthcare and not a specific proprietary business or a commercial interest.

The planning committee, staff, authors, and editors listed below have identified no financial relationships or relationships to products or devices they or their spouse/life partner have with commercial interest related to the content of this CME activity:

Amie D. Beals, PA-C; Jason Beaver, MHS, M.Ed, PA-C; Courtney L. Bennett Wilke, MPAS, PA-C; Andrea Maria Boohaker, DNP, ACNP-BC, RNFA; Larry Collins, MPAS, PA, ATC, DFAAPA; Amy Dix, PhD, PA-C; Brittany M. Dowdle; Elise Elegeert, DMSC, MS, MAT, PA-C; Victoria Gentile, PA-C, MMSc, MA; Aaron J. Guyer, MD, FAAOS; Rodney Ho, MPAS, MPH, PhD, PA-C, Psychiatry-CAQ; Katherine Holmes, MSN, APRN; Alexander Hopkins, MSPA, PA-C; Kerri Jack, MHS, PA-C; Allison J. Justice, MMS, PA-C; Alan M. Keating, MPAS, PA-C; Stephanie Kubiak, PhD, OTR/L; Kothainayaki Kulanthaivelu, BCA, MBA; Michelle Littlejohn; Amy L. Noyes, MSN, CPNP, APRN, RNFA; Kerby Pierre-Louis, MSPAS, PA-C; Susan M. Salahshor, PhD, PA-C, DFAAPA; Melissa Shaffron, DMSc, PA-C; R. Martin Shipman, Sr, MHA, PA, CMCO; Kara-Ann Valentine, MMS, PA-C; Derrick Varner, PhD, PA-C, DFAAPA, RDMS; Jodiann Williams, PA-C MSPA

UNAPPROVED/OFF-LABEL USE DISCLOSURE

The EOCME requires CME faculty to disclose to the participants:

1. When products or procedures being discussed are off-label, unlabelled, experimental, and/or investigational (not US Food and Drug Administration [FDA] approved); and
2. Any limitations on the information presented, such as data that are preliminary or that represent ongoing research, interim analyses, and/or unsupported opinions. Faculty may discuss information about pharmaceutical agents that is outside of FDA-approved labelling. This information is intended solely for CME and is not intended to promote off-label use of these medications. If you have any questions, contact the medical affairs department of the manufacturer for the most recent prescribing information.

TO ENROLL

The CME program is available to all Physician Assistant Clinics subscribers at no additional fee. To subscribe to the Physician Assistant Clinics, call customer service at 1-800-654-2452 or sign up online at www.physicianassistant.theclinics.com/.

METHOD OF PARTICIPATION

In order to claim credit, participants must complete the following:
1. Complete enrolment as indicated above
2. Read the activity
3. Complete the CME Test and Evaluation. Participants must achieve a score of 70% on the test. All CME Tests and Evaluations must be completed online

CME INQUIRIES/SPECIAL NEEDS

For all CME inquiries or special needs, please contact elsevierCME@elsevier.com.

Contributors

CONSULTING EDITORS

KIM ZUBER, PA-C
American Academy of Nephrology PAs, Melbourne, Florida

JANE S. DAVIS, BSN, MSN, DNP
Nurse Practitioner, Nephrology, The University of Alabama at Birmingham, Birmingham, Alabama

EDITOR

KARA-ANN VALENTINE, MMS, PA-C
Assistant Professor, Director of Didactic Education, Assistant Professor, School of Health Professions, Palm Beach Atlantic University, West Palm Beach, Florida

AUTHORS

AMIE D. BEALS, PA-C
Physician Assistant, Springfield Orthopaedics and Sports Medicine Institute, Springfield, Ohio

JASON BEAVER, MHS, MEd, PA-C
Assistant Professor, Florida State University College of Medicine, School of Physician Assistant Practice, Tallahassee, Florida

COURTNEY L. BENNETT WILKE, MPAS, PA-C
Physician Assistant, Tallahassee Memorial Hospital, Tallahassee, Florida

ANDREA MARIA BOOHAKER, DNP, ACNP-BC, RNFA
Advanced Practice Provider Manager, Department of Orthopaedic Surgery, The University of Alabama at Birmingham, Clinical Assistant Professor of Nursing, UAB School of Nursing at Birmingham, Birmingham, Alabama

LARRY COLLINS, MPAS, PA, ATC, DFAAPA
Associate Professor, Department of Orthopaedics and Sports Medicine, Associate Program Director, Physician Assistant Program, USF Health Morsani College of Medicine, Tampa, Florida

AMY DIX, PhD, PA-C
Cara Therapeutics, Department of Occupational Therapy, Gannon University, Erie, Pennsylvania

BRITTANY M. DOWDLE, BA
Editor/Owner, Word Cat Editorial Services, Suches, Georgia

ELISE ELEGEERT, DMSC, MS, MAT, PA-C
Assistant Professor, Florida State University College of Medicine, School of Physician Assistant Practice, Tallahassee, Florida

VICTORIA GENTILE, PA-C, MMSc, MA
Physician Assistant, Yale New Haven Health Pediatric Orthopedics, New Haven, Connecticut

AARON J. GUYER, MD, FAAOS
Clinical Assistant Professor in Surgery, Florida State University College of Medicine, Tallahassee Orthopedic Clinic, Tallahassee, Florida

RODNEY HO, MPAS, MPH, PhD, PA-C, Psychiatry-CAQ
Program Director, Rocky Mountain University, Provo, Utah

KATHERINE HOLMES, MSN, APRN
Advanced Practice Nurse, Yale New Haven Health Pediatric Orthopedics, New Haven, Connecticut

ALEXANDER HOPKINS, MSPA, PA-C
Physician Assistant, Orlando VA Medical Center, Viera Outpatient Clinic, Melbourne, Florida

KERRI JACK, MHS, PA-C
Assistant Professor/Clinical Coordinator, Chatham University PA Program, Pittsburgh, Pennsylvania

ALLISON J. JUSTICE, MMS, PA-C
Assistant Professor, Florida State University College of Medicine, School of Physician Assistant Practice, Tallahassee, Florida

ALAN M. KEATING, MPAS, PA-C, MPAS
Physician Assistant, University of Nebraska Medical Center, Omaha, Nebraska

STEPHANIE KUBIAK, PhD, OTR/L
Assistant Professor Occupational Therapy Program, Department of Occupational Therapy, Gannon University, Erie, Pennsylvania

KERBY PIERRE-LOUIS, MSPAS, PA-C
Physician Assistant, Acute Care Orthopedics, Murphysboro, Illinois

AMY L. NOYES, MSN, CPNP, APRN RNFA
Nurse Practitioner, Yale New Haven Health Pediatric Orthopedics, New Haven, Connecticut

SUSAN M. SALAHSHOR, PhD, PA-C, DFAAPA
Assistant Professor, Founding Program Director, Ithaca College Physician Assistant Program, Ithaca, New York

MELISSA SHAFFRON, DMSc, PA-C
Program Director, School of Physician Assistant Medicine, College of Medical Science, University of Lynchburg, Lynchburg, Virginia

ROBERT MARTIN SHIPMAN SR. MHA, PA, CMCO
Assistant Professor, School of Physician Assistant Practice, Florida State University College of Medicine, Tallahassee, Florida

DERRICK VARNER, PhD, PA-C, DFAAPA, RDMS
Physician Assistant, Family Medicine, Clinical Educator, San Antonio, Texas

JODIANN WILLIAMS, PA-C, MSPA
Physician Assistant, ARC Orthopedic Group, West Hills, California

Contents

> Musculoskeletal injuries and conditions are commonly seen in primary, ur-
> gent, and specialty medical clinics. The care and treatment of these types
> of conditions range from simple observation to complex, interventional,
> and surgical. Physician Associates must recognize the role that they and
> a variety of other health care providers play in the evaluation, treatment,
> management, and prevention of these injuries and conditions.

> Development and evolution of treatment plans hinge on clinical examina-
> tions and diagnostic imaging within the orthopedic subspecialty. The exe-
> cution of the appropriate imaging and accurate interpretation assists in the
> development of treatment plans and effective patient education. Although
> not always a necessity, imaging can provide clarity to a clinical presenta-
> tion or provide necessary details to formulate a treatment plan. The in-
> volvement of imaging in collaboration with physical examination
> techniques allows for more accurate differential diagnoses along with
> the initiation of the appropriate disposition.

> Upper extremity fractures and musculoskeletal disorders commonly
> present in primary care and orthopedics settings. These diagnoses can
> be associated with trauma or injury causing pain to the upper extremity,
> typically occurring secondary to falls or high-impact sports. Patients
> need evaluation and treatment to address their concerns and improve
> musculoskeletal function. This article focuses on the classification system
> of fractures and highlights fractures of the upper extremity. Each is dis-
> cussed separately with emphasis on the cause, presentation, and treat-
> ment. Acute and chronic disorders of the shoulder, elbow, and wrist are
> also described.

PHYSICIAN ASSISTANT CLINICS

SERIES OF RELATED INTEREST

Primary Care: Clinics in Office Practice
https://www.primarycare.theclinics.com/
Orthopedic Clinics
https://www.orthopedic.theclinics.com/

THE CLINICS ARE AVAILABLE ONLINE!
Access your subscription at:
www.theclinics.com

PHYSICIAN ASSISTANT CLINICS

FORTHCOMING ISSUES

April 2024
Medicine Outside Four Walls
Kim Zuber and Jane Davis, Editors

July 2024
Gender Minority Medicine
Cathe Fransen, Editor

October 2024
Advances in Patient Education: An
Inpatient Approach
Lucy W. Kibe and Gerald Kayingo, Editors

RECENT ISSUES

October 2023
Allergy, Asthma, and Immunology
Gabriel Ortiz, Editor

July 2023
Nutrition and Wellness in Medicine
Diabetes

April 2023
Dermatology
Rebecca X. Moeller, Editor

SERIES OF RELATED INTEREST

Primary Care: Clinics in Office Practice
https://www.primarycare.theclinics.com/

Dermatology
https://www.derm.theclinics.com/

Foreword

General Orthopedics

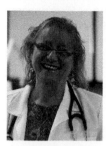 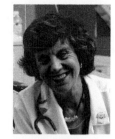

Kim Zuber, PA-C   Jane S. Davis, BSN, MSN, DNP
Consulting Editors

Sticks and stones will certainly break bones but so will falls, trauma, and a host of other events. This issue of *Physician Assistant Clinics* focuses on the structures that keep us upright and functional. Yet, when things go awry, these same bones and tissues can be painful, limit our mobility, and make us appreciate a fully functional skeleton. Most of us have had some orthopedics in our physician assistant (PA) training, but so much changes so fast. Thus, we are asking the experts to update orthopedics for us.

More than 18,000 PAs practiced orthopedics in 2022. We asked some of these experts to share their knowledge with us. And share they did! The most common complaint for a primary care visit is lower-back pain (and you thought it was the "common cold"!). So, we have the most recent data on back pain for you. None of us will get through aging without needing these ortho experts. They keep us whole, reduce our fractures, increase our mobility, and assist with activities of daily living. Orthopedics overlaps with many specialties, from primary care to nephrology to rheumatology to OB/GYN to pediatrics to neurology. There is not a specialty that doesn't share something with orthopedics. As we age, our ortho colleagues become more important, and to be honest, are now on our speed dial.

So many bones, 206 to be exact, and all working together to stand us upright and propel us through our day. The authors that Kara Valentine has gathered give us insight into what can happen to our skeletal system, from fractures to injuries to disease process and all processes in between. In these articles the reader will learn to recognize common and not so common orthopedic presentations, how to assess and how to treat and, most important, when to refer. We thank the experts for taking care of us and our patients and for sharing their insights with us all.

Physician Assist Clin 9 (2024) xiii–xiv
https://doi.org/10.1016/j.cpha.2023.09.003
2405-7991/24/© 2023 Published by Elsevier Inc.

physicianassistant.theclinics.com

Kim Zuber, PA-C
American Academy of Nephrology PAs
131 31st Avenue North
St Petersburg, FL 33704, USA

Jane S. Davis, BSN, MSN, DNP
University of Alabama at Birmingham
728 Richard Arrington Blvd S
Birmingham, AL 35233, USA

E-mail addresses:
zuberkim@yahoo.com (K. Zuber)
jsdavis@uabmc.edu (J.S. Davis)

Preface

The Body of Orthopedics 2023

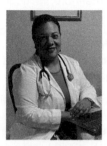

Kara-Ann Valentine, MMS, PA-C
Editor

The human body is an intricate creation with many parts partaking in various functions that are carried out by different body systems. The musculoskeletal system is one of these systems and serves to provide structure, protection, and support along with the functionality of movement. The parts of the body that assemble the musculoskeletal system include the muscles and the skeleton. The skeleton consists of bones, tendons, ligaments, and cartilage.[1] The gift of movement allows one to perform various physical activities, but this gift comes with the risk of injury. Most, if not every human being has had a musculoskeletal injury at some point in time, whether it was as minor as a simple sprained ligament of the finger or muscle contusion to as major as a compound fracture or a ruptured tendon. These injuries can occur due to trauma, misuse, or overuse, or from pathophysiologic causes. The field of orthopedics focuses on correcting and managing a musculoskeletal injury.[2] Orthopedics has several subspecialties, including pediatrics, oncology, trauma, sports medicine, and various joint specialties like hand surgery, spine surgery, total joint, and foot and ankle surgery to name a few.

The Body of Orthopedics 2023 issue informs readers about current evidence-based practices and discusses past and possible future practices. This issue touches on many of the parts that make up the body of orthopedics. First, we begin by looking at the team of interprofessional members involved in orthopedic care in "The dream team of orthopedics." Next, we review the diagnostics studies used in orthopedic practice in "Pearls for ordering and interpreting imaging in orthopedics." Then we have a series of articles based on major joints starting from the shoulder in "The upper extremity: from shoulder to wrist," the spine with "The back from top to bottom: differentials for back pain," the hip in "Hip pain: What could it mean?," to the knee with "Osteoarthritis of the Knee," and finally, "Foot and Ankle Injuries with the Rise of Pickleball." We then look at special topic areas with "Orthopedic emergencies: The Common and the Critical," "What is eating your bones? Primary bone cancers," "Numbness and Tingling, where is it coming from? A Peripheral neuropathy overview," and "Orthopedic pearls in the pediatric patient." Finally, we close the issue by reviewing the evolution of prosthetics in "Becoming Whole Again: How Prosthetics Shape the Human Experience" and predict the future of the field with "The future of orthopedics: Imagining orthopedics in the year 2100."

Every person has or will hurt themself at some point in time and will likely have to see a health care provider for some kind of musculoskeletal pain. Therefore, we hope you find this orthopedic issue informative and interesting.

I would like to thank all of the authors for their dedication and diligence. Thank you to the Elsevier staff for all of their support. Finally, thank you to the readers, both current and future practitioners, may you continue to elevate your craft with the pursuit of life-long learning and provide the highest quality of care to your patients.

Kara-Ann Valentine, MMS, PA-C
School of Health Professions
Palm Beach Atlantic University
1301 South Olive Avenue
West Palm Beach, FL 33401, USA

E-mail address:
kara_valentine@pba.edu

REFERENCES

1. Toxic Substances Portal. Health effects of exposures to substances. Available at: https://wwwn.cdc.gov/TSp/substances/ToxOrganListing.aspx?toxid=17. Accessed July 17, 2023.
2. Medline Plus. Orthopedic services. Available at: https://medlineplus.gov/ency/article/007455.htm. Accessed July 17, 2023.

The Dream Team of Orthopedics

Check for updates

Larry Collins, MPAS, PA, ATC, DFAAPA

KEYWORDS

- Orthopedic injury • Musculoskeletal injury • Orthopedic rehabilitation
- Orthopedic physician associates • Musculoskeletal health
- Musculoskeletal health care providers

KEY POINTS

- Many health care providers play important roles in preventing and caring for musculoskeletal injuries.
- Prompt and accurate diagnosis of musculoskeletal injuries and conditions is essential for successful treatment and return to normal activities.
- Physician Associates must recognize their role in the evaluation and management of musculoskeletal injuries and conditions.
- Developing and maintaining an appropriate network of referral resources optimizes patient care.

INTRODUCTION

Musculoskeletal injuries and conditions are a significant problem affecting nearly 50% of Americans over the age of 18 and almost 75% of individuals over the age of 65.[1] Injuries range from mild sprains to torn ligaments and tendons, from contusions to fractures, and from overuse disorders to chronic degenerative conditions. The care and treatment of these problems may be as simple as instructing a patient to modify activities and allow time for healing and may be as complex as requiring reconstructive surgery possibly requiring multiple procedures. As our population continues to age and the ability to stay active longer increases, these problems will only increase. Recognizing that a variety of health care providers (**Table 1**) play an important role in the care, treatment, and management of musculoskeletal injuries is essential for any practicing physician associate (PA). In many settings, PAs will play a pivotal role in the management of these conditions for their patients. When evaluating a patient with a musculoskeletal injury or disorder, PAs are trained to obtain a comprehensive history, perform a thorough physical examination, and develop a concise

Department of Orthopaedics & Sports Medicine, USF Health Morsani College of Medicine, 12901 Bruce B. Downs Boulevard MDC 5, Tampa, FL 33612-4799, USA
E-mail address: collinsl@usf.edu

Physician Assist Clin 9 (2024) 1–9
https://doi.org/10.1016/j.cpha.2023.07.004
2405-7991/24/© 2023 Elsevier Inc. All rights reserved.
physicianassistant.theclinics.com

Table 1
List of musculoskeletal health care professions

Sports Medicine Physicians	American Medical Society for Sports Medicine (AMSSM)	https://www.amssm.org/
Orthopedic Surgeons	American Academy of Orthopedic Surgeons (AAOS)	https://www.aaos.org/
Athletic Trainers	National Athletic Trainers' Association (NATA)	https://www.nata.org/
Physical Therapists	American Physical Therapy Association (APTA)	https://www.apta.org/
Occupational Therapists	American Occupational Therapy Association (AOTA)	https://www.aota.org/
Rheumatologists	American College of Rheumatology (ACR)	https://rheumatology.org/
Physical Medicine and Rehabilitation	American Academy of Physical Medicine and Rehabilitation (AAPMR)	https://www.aapmr.org/home
Pain Management Specialists	American Academy of Pain Medicine (AAMP)	https://painmed.org/
Chiropractors	American Chiropractic Association (ACA)	https://www.acatoday.org/
Podiatrists	American Podiatric Medical Association (APMA)	https://www.apma.org/
Sports Dietitian	Collegiate and Professional Sports Dietitians Association (CPSDA)	https://sportsrd.org/

differential diagnosis. This allows the PA to order and interpret appropriate imaging and laboratory testing and initiate a specific treatment plan for the patient. Understanding who and where to refer a patient for further treatment, when needed, may help avoid unnecessary health care expenses and lost time and allow for a quicker, earlier return to normal activities. Some of the health care team a PA may utilize as a referral or consultation source include the sports medicine physician, orthopedic surgeon, athletic trainer, physical therapist, occupational therapist, rheumatologist, physical medicine and rehabilitation physician, pain management specialist, chiropractor, podiatrist, and sports dietitian.

PRIMARY CARE PROVIDERS

Physicians, Pas, and advance practice nurses all care for patients throughout the lifecycle in the primary care setting. These health care providers have all completed rigorous training that should allow them to care for most common musculoskeletal conditions including sprains, strains, contusions, overuse injuries (bursitis, tendinitis), as well as degenerative conditions. Primary care providers are well-equipped to diagnose and treat these common problems enabling their patients to return to active healthy lifestyles, without unnecessary referrals. Utilizing resources in the community including local gyms, wellness and recreation centers, and programs such as Silver and Fit (https://www.silverandfit.com/) and SilverSneakers (https://tools.silversneakers.com/) may allow the health care provider to guide their patients to activities that will benefit their health and wellness. Recognizing that almost any physical activity is better than no activity and that there is no "perfect" type of exercise is important to guide patients to better health. Providers should also be aware of common fitness trends (Pickleball, HIIT, CrossFit, and so forth) and the potential injuries associated with these trends. Primary care providers must also be adept at recognizing when patients are not responding as anticipated and referring to other providers when needed.

SPORTS MEDICINE PHYSICIANS

Sports medicine physicians have completed a 1-year sports medicine fellowship after the completion of their residency. They must have completed a residency in family medicine, internal medicine, emergency medicine, pediatrics, physical medicine and rehabilitation, or osteopathic neuromusculoskeletal medicine.[2] These physicians specialize in the prevention, diagnosis, and treatment of musculoskeletal injuries and conditions that occur during physical activity. They may have a split practice as a primary care provider having a panel of primary care patients as well as treating injuries related to musculoskeletal injuries or conditions. Other sports medicine physicians practice exclusively with athletes and active individuals caring for acute and chronic musculoskeletal injuries and conditions. They may also work as part of an orthopedic or multi-specialty practice to care for the many acute non-surgical musculoskeletal conditions presenting to the clinic. These sports medicine physicians help develop treatment and rehabilitation plans for acute, chronic, and degenerative conditions. Many of these physicians also function as team physicians for sports teams, being able to care for any medical conditions of the athletes along with musculoskeletal injuries. They have close working relationships with a number of orthopedic surgical specialists in order to refer patients who require specialized interventions.

Sports medicine physicians are also commonly involved in community groups and may serve as medical directors for fitness or wellness centers. Networking with local sports medicine physicians allows the primary care provider an opportunity to stay up-to-date on activities and resources in their community that may be beneficial to their patients. These specialists also frequently conduct seminars or forums that are open to the public to inform and educate on proper ways to engage in activities that are safe and healthy.

A PA may also fill this role as a "sports medicine" PA. A PA may gain extensive experience in treating musculoskeletal conditions by working alongside a sports medicine physician or orthopedic surgeon or from previous experience as an athletic trainer or physical therapist. A PA might also gain knowledge in the treatment and management of musculoskeletal conditions through attendance at specialty conferences or seminars. A sports medicine physician or PA would be a great addition to any primary care practice to enable many non-operative musculoskeletal problems be treated on-site without the need for referral.

ORTHOPEDIC SURGEONS

Orthopedic surgeons complete 5 years of residency following medical school. Many also pursue one or more 1–2-year fellowships in a variety of areas including sports medicine, trauma, adult reconstruction, pediatrics, spine, hand, foot and ankle, musculoskeletal oncology, and shoulder/elbow. This additional training allows the orthopedic surgeon to specialize in the diagnosis, treatment, and management of musculoskeletal disorders. Orthopedic surgeons are also able to perform advanced surgical procedures to repair or reconstruct torn ligaments and tendons and fix fractured bones.

The general orthopedic surgeon has completed a 5-year residency that requires them to have clinical experiences in all orthopedic subspecialty areas (pediatrics, joint reconstruction, trauma, spine, hand, foot and ankle, sports and oncology), enabling them to have sufficient expertise as a general orthopedic surgeon. Many general orthopedic surgeons treat their patient populations in a variety of these areas. Today, most orthopedic surgeons go on to complete one or more subspecialty fellowship training program(s) following their residency that may last 1 to 2 years.[3]

The sports medicine orthopaedist specializes in the care, treatment, and management of bone and soft tissue injuries that commonly affect athletes or other active individuals. They tend to focus on the rapid diagnosis and recognition of injuries to allow a prompt return to play or work. Many of the surgeries they perform are arthroscopic to help allow for this early return. The surgeries they tend to specialize in include ligament and tendon repair and reconstruction, joint stabilization, and cartilage restoration procedures. The sports medicine orthopaedist also tends to have close working relationships with athletic trainers and physical therapists. Many of these surgeons act as team physicians for school, recreation, or professional sports teams in the community. In addition to their clinical work, they may spend several hours a week providing medical coverage at sporting events alongside athletic trainers.

Adult reconstruction specialists (also commonly known as total joint specialists) usually focus on hip and knee replacement surgery for osteoarthritis or other conditions. Some of these specialists may also perform shoulder and elbow replacement surgeries. These specialists have extensive training in not only primary joint replacements but also in revision surgery and procedures involving significant reconstruction following bone or soft tissue loss. These surgeons' practices typically include an older patient population primarily with degenerative joint disease but may include younger patients with chronic conditions or traumatic joint injuries.

Shoulder and elbow specialists are a relatively newer subspecialty. They tend to focus primarily on reconstructive procedures associated with the shoulder and elbow, including rotator cuff repair and reconstruction, shoulder replacement surgery, elbow replacement surgery, and elbow ligament reconstruction. These surgeons typically see adolescents through older adults, focusing on injuries and conditions affecting the upper extremity and primarily the shoulder and elbow.

Orthopedic spine specialists care for the entire spectrum of spine conditions, including congenital, acquired, and degenerative disorders of the cervical, thoracic, and lumbar regions. In addition to conservative, non-invasive treatments, they are trained in complex spinal instrumentation and fusion procedures that may be indicated for scoliosis or other spinal deformities. Spine specialists have close working relationships with sports medicine physicians, pain management physicians, physiatrists, and physical and occupational therapists to help focus treatment for non-surgical and postoperative patients.

Foot and ankle orthopedic specialists tend to focus on specific patient populations including traumatic foot and ankle injuries, athletes or dancers, diabetic foot complications, acquired or congenital (pediatric) deformities, and post-traumatic, degenerative, and rheumatoid foot conditions. Many of these problems may require complex treatment options that include custom-made orthosis, serial casting or splinting, reconstructive surgeries, and prolonged recovery. Foot and ankle orthopedic surgeons also perform fusions and ankle replacement procedures for degenerative and post-traumatic conditions.

Orthopedic trauma surgeons focus on acute fracture management, stabilization, and post-traumatic reconstruction. They work on all anatomic regions and their patient population may include pediatrics through the elderly. These surgeons are typically associated with large trauma hospitals or academic medical centers.

Orthopedic hand surgeons usually limit their practice to the hand and wrist, although many may extend to the elbow and even the shoulder. Hand surgeons may also have plastic surgery training allowing them to perform microvascular procedures. Most hand surgeons focus on overuse, traumatic and congenital injuries, and deformities to the hand and wrist. They will have close working relationships with occupational hand therapy specialists as well as physical therapists.

Pediatric orthopaedists focus strictly on the care of the newborn through the adolescent. They diagnose, treat and manage congenital and developmental deformities, trauma, and soft tissue injuries that are specific to this population. Many "adult" orthopaedists will not treat patients younger than 12 or 13 year old. Treatment in this population frequently involves splinting, casting, bracing, and sometimes corrective surgical procedures for alignment or limb length abnormalities. The pediatric orthopedic surgeon also performs surgical and non-surgical repairs of broken bones in this population.

Orthopedic oncologists focus on the treatment of benign and malignant tumors of the bone and soft tissues, including major reconstructive procedures. They treat all age groups, children and adults, and work closely with other oncology physicians in the care and treatment of their patients. The orthopedic oncologist is often located in an area with an academic medical center.

Orthopedic surgeons are not limited to completing one fellowship, many complete more than one subspecialty fellowship allowing them to create a unique niche for their practice. These might include trauma/shoulder/elbow, oncology/adult reconstruction, shoulder/elbow/hand, trauma/foot/ankle, and so forth.[3]

Referrals to an orthopedic surgeon are usually for musculoskeletal conditions that a PA is not experienced at evaluating and treating or a condition that will likely need surgical interventions. Common conditions might include anterior cruciate ligament tears, displaced or unstable fractures, recurrent shoulder dislocations, and osteoarthritis that has failed conservative management.

ATHLETIC TRAINERS

Athletic Trainers are specialized health care providers with extensive training in the prevention and care of medical conditions and injuries in athletes. Athletic trainers possess the knowledge and skill to provide injury and illness prevention, wellness promotion and education, basic primary care, evaluation and treatment for acute conditions, emergency care, as well as therapeutic intervention and rehabilitation of injuries and medical conditions.[4] Athletic Trainers work under the direction of or in collaboration with a physician to provide care to the population of individuals they serve.[4]

Athletic Trainers are the day-to-day health care providers for most organized competitive athletes. They can care for the daily health, injuries, and conditions that may affect the athletes under their care. This includes musculoskeletal and general health conditions. Many high schools and almost all colleges and universities employ athletic trainers as the first-line caregivers for the athletes competing at these institutions. Athletic Trainers also work in many non-sport-related settings including medical and occupational health clinics. Athletic Trainers evaluate acute and chronic injuries, develop treatment and rehabilitation plans, implement therapeutic interventions, monitor response to treatment, conduct pre-participation and injury screenings, and promote safety and injury prevention. Referrals to an athletic trainer would typically be for the rehabilitation of a sports-related injury.

PHYSICAL THERAPISTS

Physical therapists are doctoral-trained movement experts who are trained to diagnose and treat individuals of all ages with injuries, disabilities, or other health conditions through prescribed exercise, hands-on care, and patient education. Physical therapists develop personalized treatment plans that include activities and modalities designed to improve the range of motion, strength, flexibility, and function in their patients.[5] Physical therapists work in hospital and outpatient clinic settings providing hands-on care for their patients. Physical therapists may also work in medical and occupational health clinics, skilled nursing facilities, and with athletic teams. Open lines of communication between the provider, patient, and physical therapist are essential to optimizing the rehabilitation of any injury or condition. Referrals to a Physical therapist are to optimize a patient's ability to rehabilitate following an injury, trauma, or surgery. Often a physical therapist will guide the patient through a rehabilitation program until such time that the patient is able to continue rehabilitation on their own.

OCCUPATIONAL THERAPISTS

Occupational therapists are health care providers who specialize in the treatment of musculoskeletal injuries and conditions that affect an individual's ability to perform daily activities. They work closely with patients to develop personalized treatment plans that address specific functional limitations to meet goals to recover and maintain skills needed for daily and work activities. Occupational therapists utilize a range of modalities including therapeutic exercise, functional training, and adaptive equipment to help patients regain independence and improve their overall quality of life. Referral to an occupational therapist is typically to help the patient return to work or normal daily activities.

RHEUMATOLOGISTS

Rheumatologists are internal medicine or pediatric physicians who have focused training in the diagnosis, treatment, and management of diseases affecting the joints, muscles, and bones. These physicians treat systemic, immunologic, and degenerative rheumatic conditions including arthritis, back pain, and osteoporosis. Rheumatologists work closely with physical and occupational therapists, orthopaedists, neurologists, and other health care providers to deliver comprehensive care to their patients. Referrals to a rheumatologist are usually for the evaluation of patients with confirmed or suspected systemic rheumatologic conditions that fall outside the expertise of the referring provider.

PHYSICAL MEDICINE AND REHABILITATION

Physical medicine and rehabilitation physicians, also known as physiatrists, evaluate and treat patients with injuries, disorders, and disabilities of the musculoskeletal and nervous systems. This may include neck or back problems, stroke recovery, brain or spinal cord injury, spasticity, and other disabilities that impair function. Physiatrists work alongside other health care professionals to help improve the physical, mental, social, and vocational function of their patients. This includes treating pain, restoring function, and improving quality of life. Referrals to a physiatrist may be for a variety of reasons, including evaluation for neuropathies (electromyography and nerve conduction studies) and for patients requiring chronic or prolonged rehabilitation following an injury, trauma, or surgery.

PAIN MANAGEMENT SPECIALISTS

Pain management specialists are physicians who have focused their area of practice on managing acute and chronic pain in their patients. They may have trained in anesthesiology, diagnostic radiology, emergency medicine, family medicine, neurology, or physical medicine and rehabilitation and then specialized in pain management.[6] Pain management specialists diagnose and treat patients experiencing problems with acute or chronic pain, or pain related to cancer, as inpatients or outpatients and coordinate the care needs of their patients with other health care providers. These specialists may use an array of nonsurgical and complementary treatments including massage, weight loss, acupuncture, exercise, yoga, meditation, physical therapy, dietary changes, and chiropractic care. Pain management specialists also provide interventional treatments such as epidural steroid injections, nerve blocks, joint injections, radiofrequency ablation, spinal cord stimulation, or neuromodulation. PAs may consider referral to a pain management specialist for patients requiring chronic or long-term pain medications, patients requiring increasing amounts of pain medications, and patients who are not able to tolerate typical pain medication regimens.

CHIROPRACTORS

Chiropractors are trained in the diagnosis, treatment, and management of mechanical disorders of the musculoskeletal system. They must complete a doctoral-level training program that includes a minimum of 4200 instructional hours in the assessment, diagnosis, management, health promotion, and disease prevention of their patients as well as chiropractic adjustment and manipulation.[7] Chiropractors may work independently or they may partner with other health care providers (physical therapists, sports medicine physicians, orthopedic surgeons, and so forth) as part of a larger practice. They typically treat patients in independent outpatient clinical facilities or as part of larger multispecialty practices. Referrals to a chiropractor are usually for acute or chronic low-back or neck pain and as an adjuvant to physical therapy for low-back and neck problems.

PODIATRISTS

Podiatrists are doctoral-level trained health care providers who treat conditions and injuries to the foot, ankle, and related structures of the leg. Podiatrists may work independently but are often part of a larger health care practice or network, working in conjunction with orthotists, physical and occupational therapists, orthopedic surgeons, neurologists, and sports medicine physicians to provide coordinated care to patients. In the sports medicine setting referrals to a podiatrist are often for evaluation regarding orthotics or prosthetics that may be required. Podiatrists are also a great referral source for patients with chronic callus or corns, ingrown nails, and chronic nail fungus. Podiatrists are also excellent referrals for patients with diabetes mellitus who may develop peripheral neuropathies and require regular foot evaluations and maintenance.

SPORTS DIETITIAN

A Sports Dietitian is a registered dietitian who is a specialist in sports dietetics and applies evidence-based nutrition knowledge in exercise and sports. Registered dietitians specialize in assessing, educating, and counseling athletes and active individuals in nutritional plans to optimize health and well-being. The dietitian will design, implement, and manage safe and effective nutrition strategies that enhance lifelong health, fitness, and optimal performance.[8] Referral to a sports dietitian is appropriate for any patient concerned about their eating habits, who have a difficult time self-managing their diets and need guidance in developing a healthier or effective nutritional plan.

SUMMARY

PAs, and any health care provider, who provides care to patients with musculoskeletal injuries and conditions must be aware of the vital role they play in the recovery and restoration of normal function. Recognizing that they can actively work with their patients to encourage, promote and facilitate active recovery for a return to normal work and daily activities is an important part of the patient relationship. Having a network of related providers and recognizing that they each have a unique role to play in the treatment and recovery process is essential to optimizing the care provided to the patient. Developing and maintaining a close network of referral resources including orthopedic surgeons, sports medicine physicians, athletic trainers, physical and occupational therapists, chiropractors, and others is critical to having a comprehensive practice to optimize the care of your patients.

CLINICS CARE POINTS

- PAs play an integral role in the return to daily activities, play, and work for their patients diagnosed with musculoskeletal injuries or conditions.
- Recognizing that the prompt and accurate diagnosis of musculoskeletal injuries and conditions is essential for successful treatment and return to normal activities, PAs must recognize when to refer to other health care providers.
- PAs caring for patients with musculoskeletal conditions should seek to build a reliable interprofessional network that includes an array of health care providers dedicated to seeking the best possible outcomes for their patients.
- Maintaining open lines of communication between the PA, the patient, and referral sources is a key component of optimizing the management of patients with musculoskeletal conditions.

DISCLOSURE

The author has no commercial or financial conflicts of interest related to this article and no financial and/or material support was received for the creation of this article.

REFERENCES

1. United States Bone and Joint Initiative: The Burden of Musculoskeletal Diseases in the United States (BMUS), Third Edition, 2014. Rosemont, IL. Available at http://www.boneandjointburden.org. Accessed on April 8, 2023.
2. Sports Medicine: American Board of Internal Medicine. Available at: https://www.abim.org/certification/policies/internal-medicine-subspecialty-policies/sports-medicine-1/. Accessed April 21, 2023.
3. Orthopaedic Surgery Subspecialties: Accreditation Council for Graduate Medical Education (ACGME). 2000-2023. Available at https://www.acgme.org/specialties/orthopaedic-surgery/overview/. Accessed on April 24, 2023.

4. What is Athletic Training: National Athletic Trainers' Association (NATA). 2021. Available at https://www.nata.org/about/athletic-training. Accessed on April 23, 2023.
5. Becoming a PT: American Physical Therapy Association (APTA). 2023. Available at https://www.apta.org/your-career/careers-in-physical-therapy/becoming-a-pt. Accessed on April 20, 2023.
6. What is a Pain Fellowship? The Association of Pain Program Directors. https://appdhq.org/pain-fellowships/. Accessed on June 24, 2023.
7. The Council on Chiropractic Education: CCE Accreditation Standards: Principles, Processes & Requirements for Accreditation. Available at https://www.cce-usa.org/uploads/1/0/6/5/106500339/2021_cce_accreditation_standards__current_.pdf. Accessed on April 12, 2023.
8. Collegiate and Professional Sports Dietitians Association. Available at: https://sportsrd.org/. Accessed on April 19, 2023.

Pearls for Ordering and Interpreting Imaging in Orthopedics

Andrea Maria Boohaker, DNP, ACNP-BC, RNFA*

KEYWORDS

- Orthopedic imaging • Musculoskeletal imaging • Radiographs
- Orthopedic diagnostic tools

KEY POINTS

- Clinical presentation and physical examination findings should guide ordering practices to avoid unnecessary radiation risk and preventable cost to the patient.
- Appropriate selection of diagnostic imaging should be done with purpose and intention to utilize imaging to influence patient-specific treatment plans.
- Collaboration with various other subspecialties to accurately implement and interpret imaging remains imperative to effectively diagnose and begin treatment plans.

PEARLS FOR ORDERING AND INTERPRETING IMAGING IN ORTHOPEDICS

Development and evolution of treatment plans hinge on clinical examinations and diagnostic imaging within the orthopedic subspecialty. Although not always a necessity, imaging can clarify an opaque clinical presentation or provide necessary details to formulate a treatment plan.[1] The involvement of imaging as a supplement to the physical examination techniques allows for more accurate differential diagnoses along with the initiation of the appropriate disposition.[1] The execution of the appropriate imaging and accurate interpretation assists in the development of treatment plans and effective patient education.[1]

This article is not intended to discuss all possible orthopedic diagnoses and imaging options; however, it does target more commonly seen pathologies and ordering practices. If the necessity of diagnostic imaging is warranted, timely completion and cost-effectiveness should be considered to avoid any delay in treatment. Further, the involvement of various medical disciplines, such as radiology partners, can assist in ordering the most accurate test and mitigate unnecessary costs for the patient. Finally, the use of advanced diagnostic imaging should be reserved for clinical presentations

Physician Assistant Clinics- General Orthopedics, Department of Orthopedic Surgery, The University of Alabama at Birmingham
* 1313 13th Street South, Birmingham, AL 35205.
E-mail address: aboohaker@uabmc.edu

Physician Assist Clin 9 (2024) 11–18
https://doi.org/10.1016/j.cpha.2023.07.005
2405-7991/24/© 2023 Elsevier Inc. All rights reserved.
physicianassistant.theclinics.com

requiring additional information or to influence the treatment plan. Although not specific to only the orthopedic subspecialty, avoiding unnecessary radiation exposure should also influence a provider's decision to order specific diagnostic tests.[2]

RADIOGRAPHS

While considered the simplest form of diagnostic imaging, radiographs can provide a substantial amount of information regarding the patient condition and diagnosis. Radiographs are the most commonly used imaging technique to evaluate orthopedic disorders.[2] In addition to cost-effectiveness, Greenspan & Beltran[2] also reported that radiographs are timely and applicable in most orthopedic related complaints.

Radiograph interpretation should not be limited to the evaluation of bony structures and joint anatomy. To provide a thorough interpretation, soft tissue evaluation, and density changes are equally important to consider. For instance, the delineation of soft tissue involvement could indicate the presence of an open fracture, mass, or infection, which would alter the treatment course and urgency of the patient scenario.[1,2]

Plain radiographs on any joint or extremity should always include a minimum of two views, preferably three, to accurately assess the complaint. Anterior-Posterior (AP), oblique, and lateral (L) views will portray an appropriate representation of the injured structure.[2] Without the inclusion of each view, the correct diagnosis could be missed, or the incorrect treatment plan could be initiated. Delayed diagnoses or missed injuries could lead to poor outcomes and functional limitations. Along with the standard views, there are other views specific to each joint that can be utilized to assist in the diagnosis.[2]

While obtaining the appropriate views remains imperative for diagnosis purposes, some patient scenarios will require radiographs of the contralateral, uninjured extremity for comparison purposes.[1,2] The relationship between each comparison radiograph can reinforce normal anatomy versus orthopedic pathology requiring further assessment or treatment.[1] For instance, growth plate assessment in the orthopedic pediatric population is evaluated with contralateral images to determine injury or normal anatomic alignment.[1,2]

The completion of radiographs should be incorporated into each decision-making pathway when assessing orthopedic complaints. Subsequent discussion outlines specific views and applicable advanced imaging for each extremity to ensure a through radiographic evaluation. In certain scenarios, radiographs are not sufficient to develop a working diagnosis, which would warrant the involvement of advanced imaging.[1,2]

ULTRASONOGRAPHY

The cost effectiveness and versatility of ultrasonography has contributed to the overall utilization within musculoskeletal imaging.[2] Evaluation of soft tissue masses, tendon pathology, or vascular abnormalities are common reasons to incorporate an ultrasound in the treatment plan.[1] An ultrasound is an inexpensive intervention that can be used to assess tendon integrity or a soft tissue mass composition. Additionally, procedural injections or aspirations can involve the assistance of an ultrasound for accuracy and real-time evaluation of medication administration.[1]

COMPUTED TOMOGRAPHY

Advancement and sophistication of Computed Tomography (CT) technology has aided in the delineation of fracture patterns and preoperative planning. Cost inefficiencies and radiation risks remain as potential barriers for CT completion; however, the inclusion of a CT in a treatment plan should be reserved for specific patient scenarios. CT images are effective in allowing thorough the evaluation of soft tissue and articular cartilage pathology. Further, a CT can be useful to complete aspirations and bony or soft tissue biopsies.[2] Finally, if an MRI is contraindicated, a CT can be completed to provide applicable images and information.[3]

Trauma-initiated pathologies frequently benefit from the completion of CT images to quickly diagnose injuries and initiate treatment plans.[2] Through the inclusion of variable views and a variation of slice thickness, CT images are efficient and sharp with superb contrast resolution capabilities.[1] With technological developments, CT 3D reconstructions are available to further assess various anatomic areas to create precise preoperative plans.[2] Further, the ability to reformat CT images has enhanced evaluation techniques to assess alignment and orthopedic injuries.[2] Finally, CT guided biopsies are helpful for the targeted evaluation of and successful completion of bony tumors or masses.[4]

CT angiography remains another useful technique for orthopedic evaluation in certain clinical scenarios. For instance, high-energy polytrauma settings could involve the potential for a vascular injury requiring a CT angiogram. An explicit example of the aforementioned setting would include a diagnosis of scapulothoracic dissociation (STD) with a high probability of a vessel injury. A rapid assessment and recognition of a vessel injury could improve mortality and morbidity risks for STD scenarios.[5,6]

MAGNETIC RESONANT IMAGING

Despite the completion and interpretation of plain radiographs for orthopedic pathology, utilization of magnetic resonant imaging (MRI) can be useful to further develop a diagnosis and a treatment plan. Additionally, MRI imaging can assist in expounding on a clinical presentation that is difficult to diagnose. Technological advances in MRI coils have allowed for enhanced delineation of soft tissue composition and anatomic imaging. Due to cost inefficiencies, an MRI should be reserved for appropriate clinical scenarios and particular diagnoses.[1]

Orthopedic clinical presentations involving the investigation of soft tissue or bony masses should include MRI imaging for detail and diagnosis formulation.[1,2] To further characterize the disposition of a mass, an MRI achieves the goal of further classification without invasive techniques. An MRI can be a useful diagnostic tool when evaluating ligamentous integrity when developing a treatment plan. For example, an anterior cruciate ligament (ACL) evaluation should involve MRI imaging to confirm the diagnosis and implement operative or nonoperative intervention.[1,2]

An MR arthrogram is an excellent diagnostic tool for patient presentations involving joint pathologies. Indications for completing an MR arthrogram involves the suspicion for an elbow UCL injury, a wrist triangular fibrocartilage complex (TFCC) or scapholunate tear, shoulder instability pathologies, hip labral tears or femoroacetabular impingement (FAI), and postoperative meniscal evaluation in the knee.[7]

SCINTIGRAM

A bone scan utilizes a radioactive substance to help identify disease processes such as infections, fractures, or tumors.[2] Specifically, bone scans are helpful in identifying the presence of a stress fracture or an insufficiency fracture in scenarios when plain radiographs are inconclusive. Acute or chronic infections are further characterized through scintigram imaging; however, evaluation for bony metastasis is the most frequent indication for a bone scan. The images include the entire skeletal system and can utilize various contrast options dependent on the indication.[2]

IMAGING FOR SHOULDER INJURIES

Thorough clinical evaluation of shoulder pathology involves the incorporation of radiograph interpretation. In addition to AP/L/oblique views, the glenohumeral joint can be visualized through the axillary view. As one of the most frequently dislocated large joints in the body, this specialized view assists with ensuring appropriate alignment and ruling out dislocation or subluxation of the humeral head.[8] Further, the completion of scapular-Y radiographs allows for the visualization of the scapular body and spine.[3]

For patient scenarios concerned for bursitis, infection, swelling, or aspiration needs, execution of a musculoskeletal ultrasound (MSK US) can be utilized for the assessment of biceps tendon integrity, acromioclavicular (AC) joint stability, or glenohumeral joint effusions.[3] Further, ultrasound-guided injections to the shoulder are effective diagnostically and therapeutically due to the increased accuracy in the placement of the corticosteroid. Similarly, a CT can be useful in the setting of trauma for the evaluation of fracture alignment or concern for an incarcerated loose body.[1–3]

Concerns of rotator cuff or labral pathologies would indicate a need for an MRI to further evaluate the integrity of the aforementioned structures. Additionally, patients presenting with the suspicion of infection, tumors/masses, or failed conservative management would benefit from MRI imaging. Finally, an MRI is beneficial with patient scenarios involving concerns for osteonecrosis or stress fractures as these pathologies are not well defined on plain radiographs.[3]

IMAGING FOR KNEE INJURIES

Plain radiographs are designated as the first-line diagnostic tool to comprehensively evaluate the knee. Along with standard AP/L/oblique views, additional specialized views are included to better visualize all compartments of the knee.[9] Weightbearing or standing views should be included to evaluate medial and lateral compartments and will aid in identifying joint space narrowing or articular cartilage thinning.[3] Further, a sunrise view can be included to better visualize the patellofemoral juncture and can be helpful in recognizing patella subluxation. Patient presentations including generalized knee pain could benefit from the inclusion of the sunrise view.[9] Finally, an intercondylar view, also referred to as a tunnel view, allows for the assessment of the posterior portion of the femoral condyle and can identify the presence of an osteochondral lesion.[9]

Following the completion and evaluation of plain radiographs, a CT is useful in most patient scenarios involving intraarticular fracture pathology for fracture alignment or joint loose bodies.[10] In a trauma setting, tibial plateau or distal femur fractures should be further evaluated with a CT to ensure appropriate or anatomic alignment of the articular surface to assist in the prevention of poor functional outcomes or an increased risk of post-traumatic arthritis.[2,9]

Ultrasound involvement for knee pathology can be helpful in evaluating the integrity of the extensor mechanism, the presence of a localized fluid collection, or soft tissue mass. If the ultrasound is nonspecific, an MRI is indicated to further characterize a mass or delineate internal derangement for treatment initiation. An MRI will provide insight on the anatomic alignment of ligaments, tendons, menisci, and bony integrity. In specific patient settings, the use of contrast can be helpful in portraying meniscal injuries in the postoperative setting or the presence of osteochondral defects.[3]

IMAGING FOR SPINE INJURIES

Plain radiographs and CT imaging remain the mainstay techniques to assess bony structures in the spine.[11] Thorough evaluation of patients with spine complaints involves the completion of AP/L views along with specialized views in specific circumstances. Specialized views can include flexion and extension views to initially evaluate stability and alignment at each specific level.[11] If a CT is unable to be completed or unavailable, a swimmer's lateral view is necessary to adequately assess the C7 to T1 juncture. A true lateral of the spine is imperative to complete a thorough assessment of spine complaints or pathologies.[12]

A subset of spinal complaints involves a scoliosis evaluation and treatment. Diagnosis of scoliosis should involve the completion of a long plain radiograph of the entire spine. Further, lateral bending views are necessary to assess the integrity of specific curves.[13] In trauma settings, the ease of completing CT imaging has become a standard diagnostic tool for rapid diagnoses. While CT completion is necessary for comprehensive osseous evaluation in these scenarios, it should not replace plain radiography.[11] Further, procedural injections utilizing CT or ultrasound guidance is a common technique that aids in accuracy and assists in diagnostic purposes and symptomatic relief.[11]

MRI imaging should be obtained in clinical scenarios requiring detailed information on soft tissue components, spinal cord and nerve anatomy, and lesions.[11] Specific indications involve clinical presentations encompassing radiculopathy, disc herniations, autoimmune disorder concerns, infections, congenital malformations, postoperative follow-up, cervical spine fractures, and spinal hematomas or tumors.[14]

IMAGING FOR PELVIS/HIP INJURIES

Obtaining the appropriate imaging to further evaluate pelvic injuries or pathology is imperative to avoid a delay in diagnosis and treatment. At minimum, an AP pelvis and lateral should be standard of care to initially assess stability and anatomic alignment.[3] Hip diagnoses can differ depending on the patient population being evaluated. For instance, developmental dysplasia of the hip (DDH) and Legg-Calve-Perthes are common diagnoses seen in our pediatric population.[3] Additionally, evaluation of the contralateral, uninjured extremity along with radiographs of the lumbar spine allows for a thorough, all-inclusive examination for hip and pelvis complaints.[15]

Comparatively, trauma diagnoses affect the entire patient age spectrum. When a pelvic ring injury is suspected, inlet/outlet views provide the visualization of the sacrum, pubic body, and superior and inferior rami.[16,17] Further, if an acetabular fracture is suspected, judet views should be included to visualize the acetabular wall and iliac wings.[16,18] Accurate and efficient recognition of pelvic injuries allows for appropriate treatment plans to be implemented rapidly and initiation operative intervention.[17]

The completion of a CT should be considered when evaluating for a fracture pattern or assessing current state anatomy. Further, precise diagnoses such as femoroacetabular impingement (FAI) can be assessed and diagnosed through CT 3D reconstructions. Along with the diagnostic abilities of CT imaging for pelvis and hip pathologies, preoperative planning is significantly enhanced and allows for improved optimization of patient outcomes. Ultrasound involvement can be helpful in diagnostic injection scenarios for the guidance of appropriate medication placement.[15]

Soft tissue injuries, with or without intraarticular involvement, and osteonecrosis are appropriate indications for MRI completion. Degenerative disease of the pelvis/hip is also best visualized through MRI, or arthrogram imaging, which should augment suspected diagnoses from previously completed radiographs. Further, labral pathology is distinctly illustrated on MRI imaging and should be considered when formulating differential diagnoses.[15]

IMAGING FOR ANKLE/FOOT INJURIES

The ankle remains a commonly injured joint and evaluation with standard radiographs is essential. The completion of an AP, lateral, and oblique/mortise views are imperative to adequately evaluate the anatomy within the foot and ankle. Additionally, weight-bearing views can be helpful in evaluating instability and changes in anatomic alignment. If a syndesmotic, or ligamentous, injury is suspected, a stress view should be completed. A stress view adequately depicts any widening in the tibiofibular syndesmosis and the lateral and medial ligament complex.[19]

Intraarticular fractures of the foot and ankle will require CT imaging to ensure appropriate alignment and complete preoperative planning if indicated. Patients sustaining pilon fractures, talus fractures, Lisfranc injuries, calcaneal fractures, or midfoot injuries benefit from CT completion due to the spatial and 3D reconstruction capabilities for detailed evaluation.[19] Assessment of tendon pathology should utilize an MSK US or MRI imaging. For instance, Achilles tendinopathies or rupture are injuries that should involve either an ultrasound or MRI imaging to determine the most appropriate treatment plan. Further, infections, compressive neuropathies, and soft tissue masses are best evaluated with MRI images.[19]

IMAGING FOR WRIST/HAND INJURIES

Fractures, dislocations, and soft tissue injuries to the wrist can be attributed to trauma as one of the most significant causes of wrist pathologies.[20] Comprehensive understanding of wrist and hand anatomy influences decisions and treatment plans.[20] Suspicion of a wrist/hand injury should involve AP/L/oblique views prior to advanced imaging. These standard views will allow investigation to the distal radius, distal ulna, distal radioulnar joint (DRUJ), carpus, and phalanges. Despite the frequency of trauma-induced diagnoses, radiographs are also imperative in the diagnosis of osteoarthritic and rheumatologic conditions affecting the hand and wrist.[20]

Additional views that are helpful in further evaluating specific carpal bones include a scaphoid view and a clenched fist view. A scaphoid view places the hand/wrist in a deviated position to obtain a non-rotational view of distal pole, proximal pole, and waist of the scaphoid. Further, a clenched fist view should be obtained when a scapholunate ligament disruption is suspected. Both fists should be involved in a clenched fist view study to provide an accurate comparison as widening could potentially be congenital, which would not require acute treatment. If scaphoid radiographs are equivocal, a CT can easily be completed to diagnose a scaphoid fracture. If there is suspicion of scaphoid avascular necrosis, an MRI is warranted for confirmation.[20]

In the setting of swelling, concern for infection, or soft tissue mass delineation, the execution of an MSK ultrasound or MRI would be indicated. Comparatively, the completion of an MR arthrogram is necessary for the evaluation of TFCC tears, DRUJ tears, and classification of Kienbock's disease of the lunate.[2,20]

SUMMARY

The clinical examination should augment diagnostic imaging interpretation based on physical examination findings and appropriate correlation on imaging. Clinical presentation and physical examination findings should guide ordering practices to avoid unnecessary radiation risk and preventable cost to the patient. Appropriate selection of diagnostic imaging should be done with purpose and intention to utilize imaging to influence patient-specific treatment plans. As technology continues to mature, increased sophistication is inevitable with image quality and test completion for patients.

CLINICS CARE POINTS

- Radiographs are the most commonly used imaging technique to evaluate orthopedic disorders.[2]
- Radiograph interpretation should not be limited to the evaluation of bony structures and joint anatomy. To provide a thorough interpretation, soft tissue evaluation, and density changes are equally important to assess.
- Evaluation of soft tissue masses, tendon pathology, or vascular abnormalities are common reasons to incorporate an ultrasound in the treatment plan.[1] An ultrasound is an inexpensive intervention to assess tendon integrity or a soft tissue mass composition.
- CT images are effective in allowing thorough evaluation of soft tissue and articular cartilage pathology. Further, a CT can be useful to complete aspirations and bony or soft tissue biopsies.[2]
- Orthopedic clinical presentations involving the investigation of soft tissue or bony masses should include MRI imaging for detail and diagnosis formulation.[1,2]
- Indications for completing an MR arthrogram involve the suspicion for an elbow UCL injury, a wrist triangular fibrocartilage complex (TFCC) or scapholunate tear, shoulder instability pathologies, hip labral tears or FAI, and postoperative meniscal evaluation in the knee.[7]
- Bone scans are helpful in identifying the presence of a stress fracture or an insufficiency fracture in scenarios when plain radiographs are inconclusive.

DISCLOSURE

The author has no commercial or financial conflicts of interest. The author has no funding source or sources as an author.

REFERENCES

1. Pope TL, Doherty BT, Morrison WB. General imaging principles. In: Musculoskeletal imaging. 2nd edition. Philadelphia: Elsevier Saunders; 2015. p. 1–12.
2. Greenspan A, Beltran J. Imaging techniques in orthopaedics. In: Orthopaedic imaging. 7th edition. Philadelphia: Wolters Kluwer Health; 2020.
3. Mckinnis L, Mulligan ME, Duffield MA, et al. Musculoskeletal imaging handbook: a guide for primary practitioners. Philadelphia, PA: F.A. Davis Company; 2014.
4. Zurcher K, Sugi MD, Naidu SG, et al. Multimodality imaging techniques for performing challenging core biopsies. Radiographics 2020;40(3):910–1.
5. Kani K, Chew F. Scapulothoracic dissociation. Br J Radiol 2019;92(1101):20190090.
6. Choo A, Schottel P, Burgess A. scapulothoracic dissociation. J Am Acad Orthop Surg 2017;25(5):339–47.
7. Lungu E, Moser TP. A practical guide for performing arthrography under fluoroscopic or ultrasound guidance. Insights into Imaging 2015;6(6):601.
8. Foerter JA, O' Brien SD, Bui-Mansfield LT. A systemic approach to the interpretation of the shoulder radiograph to avoid common diagnostic errors. Contemp Diagn Radiol 2017;40(2):7–8.

9. De Maeseneer MO, Shahabpour M, Pope TL. Normal knee. In: Musculoskeletal imaging. 2nd edition. Philadelphia, PA: Elsevier Saunders; 2015. p. 324–32.e1.
10. Landsdown DA, Ma CB. Clinical utility of advanced imaging of the knee. J Orthop Res 2020;38(3):473–82.
11. Pressney I, Hargunani R, Khoo M, et al. Radiological imaging in the spine. Orthop Traumatol 2014;28(2):106–15.
12. Rethnam U, Yesupalan RS, Bastawrous SS. The swimmer's view: does it really show what it is supposed to show? A retrospective study. BMC Med Imag 2008;8(1):2.
13. Kim H, Kim SK, Moon ES, et al. Scoliosis imaging: what radiologists should know. Radiographics 2010;30(7):1823–42.
14. Vargas M, Boto J, Meling T. Imaging of the spine and spinal cord: An overview of magnetic resonance imaging (MRI) techniques. Revue Neurlogique 2021;177(5): 451–8.
15. Lad N, Kropf EJ. Hip pathology evaluation and imaging. Operat Tech Orthop 2019;29(4):100734.
16. Hutt JR, Ortega-Briones A, Daurka JS, et al. The ongoing relevance of acetabular fracture classification. Bone Joint Lett J 2015;97-B(8):1139–43.
17. Young JW, Burgess AW, Brumback RJ, et al. Pelvic fractures: value of plain radiography in early assessment and management. Radiology 1986;160(2):445–51.
18. Saterbak AM, Marsh JL, Turbett T, et al. Acetabular fractures classification of Letournel and Judet—a systematic approach. Iowa Orthop J 1995;15:184–96.
19. Doody O, Hopper MA. Imaging of the foot and ankle. Orthop Traumatol 2014; 28(5):339–49.
20. Heire P, Temperley D, Murali R. Radiological imaging of the wrist joint. Orthop Traumatol 2017;31(4):248–56.

The Upper Extremity
From Shoulder to Wrist

Melissa Shaffron, DMSc, PA-C

KEYWORDS

- Orthopedics • Upper extremity disorders • Fracture classification
- Shoulder disorders • Elbow disorders • Wrist disorders

KEY POINTS

- Fractures are classified by standardized terminology depicting the fracture location, morphology, and descriptive modifiers.
- Upper extremity fractures are common, typically occurring secondary to falls or high-impact sports.
- Displaced or dislocated fractures impacting joint function are indications for surgical fixation.
- Repetitive, overuse disorders of the upper extremity are treated conservatively with NSAIDs and decreased use of the joint before corticosteroids and surgical intervention are considered.
- History and physical examination are often diagnostic for upper extremity disorders.

FRACTURES
Classification

When a bone fracture occurs, it is described and documented using the fracture and dislocation classification developed by the Orthopedic Trauma Association.[1] This classification assists with the standardization of terminology and ensures communication between health care professionals is consistent when discussing a fracture. It also serves as a treatment and prognosis guide for ways a fracture can present. The classification consists of defining the bone fractured and then depicting the fracture location, morphology, and additional modifiers. If one bone has two fractures, each fracture is classified separately.[1,2]

Fracture location
Each bone has a proximal end segment, diaphysis segment, and distal end segment. Fracture location is determined by where the center of the fracture is present on the bone (**Fig. 1**).[1,2]

School of PA Medicine, College of Medical Science, University of Lynchburg, 1501 Lakeside Drive, Lynchburg, VA 24501, USA
E-mail address: shaffron_mj@lynchburg.edu

Physician Assist Clin 9 (2024) 19–31
https://doi.org/10.1016/j.cpha.2023.07.006
2405-7991/24/© 2023 Elsevier Inc. All rights reserved.
physicianassistant.theclinics.com

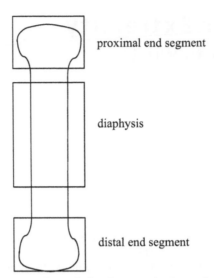

proximal end segment

diaphysis

distal end segment

Fig. 1. Fracture location. Location of the fracture is determined to be proximal end segment, diaphysis, or distal end segment.[1,2]

Fracture morphology
The morphology of the fracture is based on the location, fracture type, and fracture pattern. Diaphyseal and end segment fractures are separated into:[1,2]

- Diaphyseal (**Fig. 2**)
  - Simple: single circumferential complete fracture
  - Wedge: main fracture fragments that connect
  - Multifragmentary: multiple fracture fragments and lines
- End segment (**Fig. 3**)

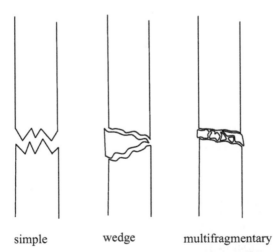

simple   wedge   multifragmentary

Fig. 2. Diaphyseal types. Define diaphyseal fractures by simple, wedge, or multifragmentary patterns.[1,2]

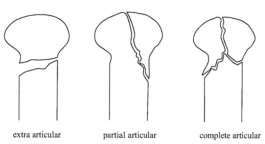

extra articular   partial articular   complete articular

Fig. 3. End segmental types. Define end segmental fractures by extra-articular, partial articular, or complete articular involvement.[1,2]

- o Extra-articular: fracture present at proximal or distal end segment but does not involve the articular surface of the bone
- o Partial articular: fracture involves some of the articular surface, but the remainder of the end segment is intact with the diaphyseal
- o Complete articular: fracture through the articular surface and the end segment, completely separating the articular surface from the diaphyseal

The fracture types separate into fracture patterns (**Table 1**).[1,2]

Fracture modifiers

Modifiers are descriptive terms that provide additional details about the fracture. The modifiers commonly used are:[1,2]

- Displaced/nondisplaced
  - o Loss of alignment between fracture and bone along the long axis
- Impaction/no impaction

Table 1
Fracture classification

Fracture Location	Fracture Type	Fracture Pattern
Diaphyseal	Simple	Spiral
		Oblique
		Transverse
	Wedge	Intact wedge
		Fragmented wedge
	Multifragmentary	Intact segmental
		Fragmentary segmental
End segment	Extra-articular	Avulsion
		Simple
		Wedge
		Multifragmentary
	Partial articular	Simple
		Split and/or depression
		Multifragmentary
	Complete articular	Simple articular with simple metaphyseal
		Simple articular with multifragmented metaphyseal
		Multifragmented articular with multifragmented metaphyseal

Determine the fracture pattern based on fracture location and fracture type.[1,2]

- ○ Compression of the fractured bone
- Dislocation
  - ○ Loss of alignment of the fracture fragment
    - ■ Anterior, posterior, medial, lateral, inferior, or multidirectional
- Open/closed fracture
  - ○ Disruption of soft tissue and potential exposure to the environment

Clavicular Fracture

Fractures of the clavicle account for 2% to 10% of all fractures, occurring more commonly in childhood and elderly populations.[3] Midshaft diaphyseal fractures represent most clavicular fractures secondary to falls and sports injuries.[3,4] Distal end segment fractures are less common and correlate with falls in the elderly population.[5]

Presentation

Pain to the fracture site following a fall or direct injury is the most common symptom. On physical examination, there may be edema, ecchymosis, or crepitus with localized tenderness to the fracture site. Complete a neurovascular examination of the extremity to evaluate for brachial plexus and subclavian vessel injury.[3] Decreased sensation and muscle weakness are associated with brachial plexus involvement. Decreased distal pulses are indicative of subclavian vessel injury.[3]

Diagnosis/imaging

Radiograph of the clavicle with anteroposterior (AP) and 45° cephalic tilt views is the standard for diagnosis. If distal or proximal end segment fracture is present, use a computed tomography of the clavicle to evaluate and guide treatment.[3]

Treatment

Conservative nonoperative management is the most common approach to clavicle fracture. Immobilization with a sling and analgesics as needed for 6 weeks is the gold standard for proximal segment and midshaft fractures.[3–5] If the fracture is at the distal end segment, refer to an orthopedic specialist for consideration of surgical treatment because of elevated risk of nonunion.[4] If suspicious of brachial plexus subclavian vessel injury, immediately consult an orthopedic specialist.[3]

Scapular Fracture

Scapular fractures are rare and account for 1% of all fractures, occurring more frequently in men between 20 and 50 years old.[6] The cause of most scapular fractures is high-energy trauma, such as motor vehicle accident, fall from height, or direct trauma to the shoulder.

Presentation

Patients present with a history of trauma or injury to the shoulder with associated pain to the region. The physical examination elicits pain during the range of motion of the shoulder joint and tenderness to palpation of the scapula with potential ecchymosis and edema.[6]

Diagnosis/imaging

Initial diagnosis occurs by AP, axial, and scapular lateral radiograph views of the shoulder. Further imaging with a computed tomography of the shoulder occurs if surgical treatment is required.[6]

Treatment

Nondisplaced scapular fractures are treated conservatively with immobilization and analgesics. Displaced fracture with concern for decreased function of the glenohumeral or scapulothoracic joint should lead one to consider surgical fixation.[6]

Humeral Fracture

Humerus fractures are the third most common fracture in the elderly population and typically occur because of low-energy falls.[7] Because of the mechanism of low-energy falls, the proximal humerus is typically fractured. In younger patients, fractures occur because of high-energy injuries, with the highest incidents of fractures located at the midshaft diaphysis.[7,8]

Presentation

A history of falls or injury with pain over the upper arm is a typical presentation for humerus fractures. A patient can experience decreased range of motion of the shoulder and/or elbow joint depending on the fracture location.[8] Tenderness over the fracture site is present with or without ecchymosis and edema. Deformity overlying fracture location is common.[8]

Diagnosis/imaging

Lateral and AP views of the humerus with a radiograph is the diagnostic standard.[8]

Treatment

Treatment of nondisplaced fractures occurs with immobilization via a long arm splint initially. After 2 weeks, the patient should be placed in an upper arm functional brace, stabilizing the fracture and allowing for movement of the shoulder and elbow joints.[8] If the fracture is displaced or nonunion occurs, surgical intervention via open reduction and internal fixation is indicated.[8]

Radius Fracture

Fractures to the proximal end segment of the radius are referred to as radial head fractures and occur because of direct elbow trauma or falling on an outstretched hand.[9] Distal radius fractures are the most common upper extremity injury, occurring when falling on an outstretched hand.[10] When the radius is fractured at the distal end segment and has dorsal comminution, dorsal angulation, dorsal displacement, and radial displacement, it is referred to as a Colles fracture.[11]

Presentation

Presentation is with pain to the forearm, elbow, or wrist after fall or direct trauma. Physical examination shows tenderness to palpation of fracture location and overlying edema.[10,11] Decreased range of motion to the elbow or wrist, dependent on the location of the radius fracture, can occur.

Diagnosis/imaging

Suspicion of fracture at the distal end segment warrants a radiograph of the wrist in AP, lateral, and oblique views.[10,11] Fractures to the proximal end segment or shaft of the radius warrant radiograph of the forearm in AP and lateral views.

Treatment

Distal radius fractures are treated acutely with immobilization via a sugar tong splint and analgesics. Most distal radius and Colles fractures are treated conservatively with cast placement for 6 weeks.[10,11] If a displaced fracture slows healing or function of the joint, reduction or surgical intervention may be considered.[10]

Proximal radius fractures are treated acutely with immobilization via a long arm splint and analgesics.[9] An aligned fracture is immobilized for 2 weeks with early range of motion of the elbow joint. Comminuted or displacement of the fracture may require elbow arthroscopy or surgical reduction with internal fixation.[9]

Ulna Fracture

Fracture to the distal ulna is associated with a distal radius fracture in 40% of cases.[12] As with radius fractures, ulna fractures occur secondary to falling on an outstretched hand.[13]

Presentation
History and physical examination are similar to radius fractures. Palpation elicits pain in the fracture location. A deformity may be visualized.[13]

Diagnosis/imaging
A suspected fracture at the distal end segment warrants a radiograph of the wrist in AP, lateral, and oblique views. Fractures to the proximal end segment or shaft of the ulna are diagnosed with a radiograph of the forearm in AP and lateral views.[13]

Treatment
Distal ulna fractures are treated with immobilization via a sugar tong splint because of the frequency associated with a fracture to the distal radius. Most fractures are treated conservatively with cast placement for 6 weeks.[12]

Proximal ulna fractures are immobilized with a long arm splint at the initial diagnosis.[14] Reevaluate in 2 weeks to determine the length of continued splint placement. If dislocation or decreased elbow joint function are present, surgery to reduce and internally fixate may be indicated.[14]

Scaphoid Fracture

Scaphoid fractures account for 60% to 70% of all carpal fractures and occur frequently with high-impact sports when falling on an outstretched hand.[15]

Presentation
Patients present with pain in the wrist after trauma or fall. Tenderness to the anatomic snuffbox increases suspicion of scaphoid fracture.[15] The patient may also have edema, decreased range of motion, and weakness during grip strength.

Diagnosis/imaging
Imaging with a radiograph of the wrist and scaphoid in posteroanterior (PA), lateral, oblique, and angled PA views are indicated. Because of the rate of missed scaphoid fractures with initial imaging, repeat radiograph in 2 weeks if symptoms persist is standard.[15] Further evaluation with MRI is also a consideration.

Treatment
Thumb spica splint for confirmed and highly suspected scaphoid fracture is acute treatment. Reevaluation and confirmation of fracture on repeat imaging calls for treatment with a cast or brace for 6 to 12 weeks.[15] Displaced fractures may indicate the need for surgical treatment.

Metacarpal Fracture

Fracture to a metacarpal is a common injury, typically occurring with direct trauma.[16] One or multiple metacarpals can be fractured, depending on the inciting trauma. The fifth metacarpal is the most commonly fractured and is also known as a "Boxer's fracture," because of the incidence of fracture associated with punching an object.[16]

Presentation
A history of direct trauma to the hand or punching an object can raise suspicion of metacarpal fracture. Patients have point tenderness to the fracture site with edema, decreased grip strength, and possible deformity.[16]

Diagnosis/imaging
Imaging with a radiograph of the hand in PA, lateral, and oblique views is diagnostic of metacarpal fracture.[16]

Treatment
Conservative treatment with a volar or ulnar gutter splint followed by cast placement for 6 weeks is standard for nondisplaced or minimally displaced fractures.[16] If the fracture is significantly displaced, caused loss of height to the metacarpal bone, or will interfere with the function of the hand, surgery with reduction and internal fixation is indicated.[16]

Phalanx Fracture

Phalanx fractures occur in all age groups but are more common in younger patients because of participation in sports and physical activities.[17] Fractures are caused by direct trauma, twisting, or crushing injury.

Presentation
Patients present with a history of injury and pain to a phalanx. The physical examination elicits tenderness to the phalanx with edema and decreased range of motion is present.[17] Deformity, ecchymosis, and paresthesia may also be appreciated.

Diagnosis/imaging
Radiograph of the affected digit in PA, lateral, and oblique views confirms the diagnosis.[17]

Treatment
Most phalanx fractures are treated conservatively with immobilization via splint for 2 to 4 weeks.[17] Intra-articular or severely displaced fractures warrant surgical intervention to reduce fracture, stabilize with fixation, and preserve digit function.

SHOULDER DISORDERS
Rotator Cuff Tear

Acute or chronic injury can cause a rotator cuff tear.[18] Acute causes include falls or a sudden pull on the arm placing strain on the shoulder muscles. Repetitive overhead or lifting movements risk leading to chronic injury and rotator cuff tear.

Presentation
Patients present with pain in the shoulder, worsening with overhead movements. Nocturnal pain is classic.[18] Muscle strength testing should be performed on the following muscles: supraspinatus, infraspinatus, teres minor, and subscapularis. Patients with pain only during a strength test are likely to have a partial tear. Patients with pain and weakness could have a complete tear of the muscle. Rotator cuff tear can cause impingement syndrome presenting similarly with positive Neer and Hawkins impingement tests.[18]

Diagnosis/imaging
MRI of the shoulder is the gold standard for confirming rotator cuff tears.[18] Radiographs to rule out other differentials may be warranted.

Treatment
Partial rotator cuff tears should be treated with physical therapy, allowing the tear to heal and strengthening the muscles.[18] Full thickness tears worsen with time and typically require surgical fixation.

Impingement Syndrome

Impingement syndrome is caused by rotator cuff tears, bursitis, bone spurs, muscle imbalance, or other disorders causing inflammation of the shoulder.[18]

Presentation
Pain worse at night and with overhead movements are hallmarks of impingement syndrome. Patients may also have pain with internal rotation to the shoulder and tenderness to palpation of the anterolateral shoulder.[18] Neer and Hawkins impingement tests elicit pain. If a rotator cuff tear is present, weakness may be appreciated.

Diagnosis/imaging
MRI of the shoulder can diagnose underlying cause contributing to impingement syndrome.[18] Shoulder radiograph should be obtained to rule out other acute differentials.

Treatment
Physical therapy to strengthen the rotator cuff muscles and avoidance of activities increasing inflammation of the shoulder girdle are first-line treatment.[18] Symptoms persisting or muscle weakness noted on physical examination indicate surgical intervention is needed to address impingement cause.

Adhesive Capsulitis

Adhesive capsulitis is an acute inflammation of the shoulder capsule leading to scarring and a frozen shoulder.[18] The cause of the acute inflammation can be trauma, surgery, or no known inciting injury may be noted. Perimenopausal women and patients with diabetes mellitus have a higher incidence rate of adhesive capsulitis.[18]

Presentation
Adhesive capsulitis has three phases within the disease process: (1) inflammatory, (2) freezing, and (3) thawing.[18] The inflammatory phase begins and progresses over 4 to 6 months with increasing inflammation of the shoulder capsule.[18] Patients present with worsening shoulder pain and limited range of motion to the joint. Assessment during this phase has decreased active and passive range of motion and limited external rotation of the shoulder with the elbow at the trunk.

The freezing phase follows with an improvement of shoulder pain, despite the continuation of a limited range of motion.[18] Physical examination has worsened active and passive range of motion than previously noted in the inflammatory phase. This phase lasts 4 to 6 months.[18]

The last phase is the thawing phase.[18] Patients have little to no shoulder pain and an improved range of motion to the shoulder joint. Assessment over 1 year have increasing active and passive range of motion. The complete course of adhesive capsulitis is 20 to 24 months.[18]

Diagnosis/imaging

Shoulder radiograph to rule out other differentials is considered; however, adhesive capsulitis typically is a clinical diagnosis.[18]

Treatment

Nonsteroidal anti-inflammatory drugs (NSAIDs) and physical therapy during the inflammatory and freezing phases are the treatments of choice.[18] This improves pain and preserves the motion of the shoulder joint. Without continued movement and physical therapy, the range of motion decreases significantly. Treatment with oral prednisone and intra-articular corticosteroid injection have shown short-term improved pain without long-term improved range of motion.[18]

Biceps Tendon Rupture

Rupture of the biceps tendon can occur in either the proximal or distal aspect of the muscle. Proximal rupture is more common and typically involves the proximal long head tendon.[19] Mechanism of proximal rupture is sudden or prolonged contraction of the biceps against resistance with the elbow flexed. Distal rupture is caused by a sudden biceps extension against resistance with the elbow extended.

Presentation

Rupture of the proximal biceps tendon presents with pain in the anterior shoulder and possibly recall of a pop or snap when the injury occurred.[19] Edema and tenderness to palpation of the bicipital groove is present. Ecchymosis may be present on the anterior upper arm. Flexion of the elbow causes pain and a "pop eye" deformity to the midarm caused by biceps muscle contracting without the resistance of the proximal tendon.[19]

Rupture to the distal biceps causes pain in the antecubital fossa.[19] Edema and tenderness to palpation in the antecubital fossa are present. The biceps squeeze test does not cause supination of the forearm and indicates distal rupture has occurred.

Diagnosis/imaging

Because of the risk of avulsion fracture, radiograph of the shoulder or elbow should be performed.[19] Ultrasound of the affected tendon can help determine a partial or complete rupture; however, an MRI of the biceps is most diagnostic.[20]

Treatment

Conservative management for proximal biceps tendon rupture and distal biceps tendon rupture affecting less than 50% of the tendon is the gold standard.[19,20] Patients should use a shoulder sling or shoulder-arm immobilizer for up to 3 weeks.[20] Early range of motion and physical therapy allows for healing and strengthening of the biceps muscle.[19]

Complete or partial tendon rupture affecting more than 50% of the tendon requires surgery to repair and reattach the tendon, restoring the function of the muscle.[20]

ELBOW DISORDERS
Lateral Epicondylitis

Lateral epicondylitis, "tennis elbow," is caused by inflammation and overuse of the wrist extensor muscles, most commonly the extensor carpi radialis brevis.[21] The diagnosis is often made in tennis players and manual workers caused by repetitive overuse of forearm muscles to extend the wrist.

Presentation

Patients present with pain to the lateral elbow and possible radiation of discomfort to the distal forearm.[21] Point tenderness to the lateral epicondyle and proximal lateral forearm muscles is diagnostic. Pain elicited with wrist extension against resistance to the lateral epicondyle, referred to as the Thomsen test, is positive.[21]

Diagnosis/imaging

AP and lateral radiographs of the elbow are ordered to rule out other differentials.[21]

Treatment

Discontinuation of repetitive movements, physical therapy for the forearm muscles, and NSAIDs are the treatment of choice for lateral epicondylitis.[21] Corticosteroid injection is considered if initial treatment fails and is found to provide relief of symptoms for several weeks.

Medial Epicondylitis

Medial epicondylitis is caused by inflammation and overuse of the wrist flexor muscles.[22] Baseball players, golfers, carpenters, and plumbers are predisposed to this diagnosis.

Presentation

Pain to the medial aspect of the elbow is the typical presenting feature. During an assessment, the patient has point tenderness to the medial epicondyle and proximal medial forearm muscles.[22] Wrist flexion against resistance produces pain at the medial elbow.

Diagnosis/imaging

AP and lateral radiographs of the elbow should be ordered to rule out other differentials.[22]

Treatment

Anti-inflammatory drugs, such as NSAIDs, physical therapy for the forearm muscles, and reduction of repetitive wrist flexion are the treatment of choice.[22] Injection with corticosteroids is warranted if improvement of symptoms with conservative treatment fails.

Olecranon Bursitis

Olecranon bursitis is an increase in fluid within the bursa cavity.[23] This is caused by trauma; inflammation; infection (septic bursitis); or underlying medical conditions, including rheumatoid arthritis and gout. The most common cause is repetitive overuse of the elbow joint and direct repetitive pressure to the bursa.

Presentation

Patients present with swelling and pain at the elbow overlying the olecranon bursa.[23] The severity of pain depends on the amount of fluid within the bursa and the underlying cause. Inflammatory causes have minimal to moderate pain, enlargement of the olecranon bursa with tenderness to palpation, and minimal surrounding edema.[24] Active and passive range of motion is intact. Infectious causes have moderate to severe pain, enlargement of the olecranon bursa with tenderness to palpation, and overlying erythema with warmth to the skin. A limited range of motion of the elbow is also present.

Diagnosis/imaging
If trauma has occurred to the elbow, radiograph with AP and lateral views are indicated to rule out a fracture or foreign body.[24] Synovial fluid aspiration with Gram stain, culture, crystal analysis, and cell count is called for if concerned for infectious cause.[24]

Treatment
Inflammatory and traumatic olecranon bursitis is managed with compression via ace wrap, NSAIDs, and decreased use of the elbow joint.[23] Corticosteroid injection of the bursa does not significantly improve outcomes, and can unnecessarily expose patients to a risk of infection.[24] Septic bursitis should be started on broad-spectrum antibiotics immediately after aspiration occurs.[23,24] If the infection is mild, outpatient treatment with oral antibiotics and close follow-up is appropriate. Moderate to severe infections should be hospitalized with intravenous antibiotics and possible open drainage procedures.[23]

WRIST/HAND DISORDERS
Carpal Tunnel Syndrome

Carpal tunnel syndrome is caused by compression of the median nerve as it passes through the carpal tunnel of the wrist.[25] Risk factors for developing carpal tunnel syndrome include pregnancy, endocrine disorders, and female gender. Overuse of the wrist causing inflammation of the carpal tunnel can also occur.

Presentation
Acute carpal tunnel syndrome presents with pain to the palmar wrist and numbness distribution of the median nerve (thumb, index, middle, and radial half of ring fingers).[25] Symptoms may worsen at night or with increased flexion and extension activities of the affected wrist. Chronic carpal tunnel syndrome presents similarly to acute but with a history of symptoms for an extended amount of time and numbness of fingers lasting longer throughout the day.[25] Physical examination may note decreased sensation to median nerve distribution of fingers, and if chronically, severe atrophy of thenar muscles and decreased pinch and grip strength may be present. Tinel sign (wrist extension test) and Phalen sign (wrist flexion test) elicit worsening of pain and numbness and assist with confirming the diagnosis.

Diagnosis/imaging
Carpal tunnel syndrome is a clinical diagnosis; however, electromyography and nerve conduction studies are indicated in some patients.[25] These additional tests are typically reserved for patients not improving with conservative treatment and surgical management is needed.

Treatment
The first-line treatment of acute carpal tunnel syndrome is a wrist splint and NSAIDs.[25] Patients should be counseled to wear the splint during activities and at night while sleeping. Patients with chronic carpal tunnel are recommended to continue use of the wrist splint in addition to a corticosteroid injection. Surgical treatment with carpal tunnel release is performed if nonsurgical options have not improved symptoms.[25]

De Quervain Tenosynovitis

The dorsal compartment of the wrist, similar to the carpal compartment, is prone to inflammatory changes leading to de Quervain tenosynovitis.[26] Overuse of the abductor pollicis longus and the extensor pollicis brevis causes inflammation of the associated tendons as they pass through the dorsal compartment. Such activities as golfing and playing video games are prone to de Quervain tenosynovitis.

Presentation
Patients present with pain at the radial aspect of the wrist near the radial styloid.[26] Tenderness to palpation of the radial lateral wrist near the dorsal compartment is present. Finkelstein test, thumb flexion against the palm with a closed fist, and ulnar deviation of the wrist elicit pain and are diagnostic.

Diagnosis/imaging
Clinical diagnosis with history and physical examination does not require further imaging.[26]

Treatment
Conservative management with NSAIDs and thumb spica splint typically resolves symptoms.[26] If pain persists, corticosteroid injections are used. Surgical release of the dorsal compartment is indicated if other treatments fail and pain persists.

CLINICS CARE POINTS

- Distal radial fractures are the most common injury of the upper extremity and should be treated with acute immobilization via a sugar tong splint and cast placement at reevaluation for 4 to 6 weeks.

- Partial rotator cuff tear results in pain to muscle strength testing with preserved muscle strength, whereas complete rotator cuff tear has pain and decreased muscle strength on physical examination.

- Adhesive capsulitis has a course of disease lasting 20 to 24 months with NSAIDs and physical therapy as treatments of choice.

- Repetitive use of wrist flexors can lead to medial epicondylitis, whereas repetitive use of wrist extensors can lead to lateral epicondylitis. Both disorders are treated first line with NSAIDs and decreased use of wrist and forearm muscles.

- History and physical examination of olecranon bursitis distinguish between inflammatory and infectious cause, guiding the treatment plan.

- The median nerve travels through the carpal compartment and distributes to the thumb, index, middle, and radial ring finger. Numbness and decreased sensation to this distribution is diagnostic for carpal tunnel syndrome.

DISCLOSURE

The author has nothing to disclose.

REFERENCES

1. Meinberg EG, Agel J, Roberts CS, et al. Fracture and dislocation classification compendium-2018. J Orthop Trauma 2018;32(Suppl 1):S1–170.
2. Karam MD, Marsh JL. Classification of fractures. In: Tornetta P, Ricci WM, Ostrum RF, et al, editors. Rockwood and green's fractures in adults. 9th edition. Philadelphia: Wolters Kluwer; 2020. p. 104–22.
3. Bentley TP, Hosseinzadeh S. In: StatPearls, editor. Clavicle fractures. 2022. Available at: https://www.ncbi.nlm.nih.gov/books/NBK507892/. Accessed April 8, 2023.

4. Moverly R, Little N, Gulihar A, et al. Current concepts in the management of clavicle fractures. J Clin Orthop Trauma 2020;11(1):S25–30.

5. Kim DW, Kim DH, Kim BS, et al. Current concepts for classification and treatment of distal clavicle fractures. Clin Orthop Surg 2020;12(2):135–44.

6. Limb D. Scapula fractures: a review. EFORT Open Rev 2021;6(6):518–25.

7. Brorson S, Palm H. Proximal humeral fractures: the choice of treatment. In: Falaschi P, Marsh D, editors. Orthogeriatrics: the management of older patients with fragility fractures. 2nd edition. Cham: Springer; 2020. p. 143–53.

8. Gallusser N, Barimani B, Vauclair F. Humeral shaft fractures. EFORT Open Rev 2021;6(1):24–34.

9. Van Riet RP, Van Den Bekerom MP, Van Tongel A, et al. Radial head fractures. Shoulder Elbow 2020;12(3):212–23.

10. Cognet JM, Mares O. Distal radius malunion in adults. Orthop Traumatol-Sur 2021;107(1). https://doi.org/10.1016/j.otsr.2020.102755.

11. Panigrahi TK, Ray S, Mallik M, et al. Determining the borderline anatomical parameters for better functional outcome of Colles fracture: a prospective study. Rev Bras Ortop (Sao Paulo) 2021;57(4):619–28.

12. Logan AJ, Lindau TR. The management of distal ulnar fractures in adults: a review of the literature and recommendations for treatment. Strategies Trauma Limb Reconstr 2008;3(2):49–56.

13. Fish MJ, Palazzo M. In: StatPearls, editor. Distal ulnar fractures. 2022. Available at. https://www.ncbi.nlm.nih.gov/books/NBK580565/. Accessed on April 8, 2023.

14. Duparc F, Merlet MC. Prevention and management of early treatment failures in elbow injuries. Orthop Traumatol Surg Res 2019;105(1S):S75–87.

15. Clementson M, Bjorkman A, Thomsen NO. Acute scaphoid fractures: guidelines for diagnosis and treatment. EFORT Open Rev 2020;5(2):96–103.

16. Carreno A, Ansari MT, Malhotra R. Management of metacarpal fractures. J Clin Orthop Trauma 2020;11(4):554–61.

17. Kremer L, Frank J, Lustenberger T, et al. Epidemiology and treatment of phalangeal fractures: conservative treatment is the predominant therapeutic concept. Eur J Trauma Emerg Surg 2022;48(1):567–71.

18. Luke A, Ma C. Musculoskeletal injuries of the shoulder. In: Papadakis MA, McPhee SJ, Rabow MW, et al, editors. Current medical diagnosis & treatment 2023. 62nd edition. USA: McGraw Hill; 2023. p. 1678–90.

19. Chow YC, Lee SW. Elbow and forearm injuries. In: Tintinalli JE, Ma O, Yealy DM, et al, editors. Tintinalli's emergency medicine: a comprehensive study guide, 9e. McGraw Hill; 2020. Available at: https://accessmedicine-mhmedical-com.ezproxy.lynchburg.edu/content.aspx?bookid=2353&sectionid=222324767. Accessed April 13, 2023.

20. Vishwanathan K, Soni K. Distal biceps rupture: evaluation and management. J Clin Orthop Trauma 2021;19:132–8.

21. Lenoir H, Mares O, Carlier Y. Management of lateral epicondylitis. Orthop Traumatol Surg Res 2019;105(8):S241–6.

22. Barco R, Antuña SA. Medial elbow pain. EFORT Open Rev 2017;2(8):362–71.

23. Blackwell JR, Hay BA, Bolt AM, et al. Olecranon bursitis: a systematic overview. Shoulder Elbow 2014;6(3):182–90.

24. Khodaee M. Common superficial bursitis. Am Fam Physician 2017;95(4):224–31.

25. Wright AR, Atkinson RE. Carpal tunnel syndrome: an update for the primary care physician. Hawaii J Health Soc Welf 2019;78(11 Suppl 2):6–10.

26. Goel R, Abzug JM. De Quervain's tenosynovitis: a review of the rehabilitative options. Hand (N Y) 2015;10(1):1–5.

The Back from Top to Bottom
Differentials for Back Pain

Susan M. Salahshor, PhD, PA-C, DFAAPA

KEYWORDS

- Back pain • Low back pain • Acute back pain • Chronic back pain
- Nonspecific back pain • Disabling • Biopsychosocial framework

KEY POINTS

- The thorough, focused, and comprehensive history and physical examination remains key to developing a differential diagnosis list for the causes of back pain.
- Clinicians must be able to recognize the red flags and alarm symptoms of back pain that require immediate attention and referral.
- Application of a biopsychosocial approach is critical to alleviating the burden of back pain for patients.
- Management of back pain requires a team approach to improve health outcomes for patients.

INTRODUCTION

The differential diagnosis of back pain is a source of frustration, challenge, and complexity for clinicians in primary care and beyond. In the global landscape, low back pain (LBP) is burdensome, costly (economically and psychosocially), and leads to disability.[1–4] The Centers for Disease Control and Prevention stated LBP has the highest prevalence of pain in the spine.[5] Therefore, gathering the history, performing a focused and comprehensive physical examination, and choosing the right diagnostic tools are paramount in primary care to enable clinicians to treat their patients and determine when to refer them.

History

The first report of backache (hereafter referred to as back pain) was in 1500 BC by an Egyptian scribe.[6] At that time, the written information did not give a diagnosis or state the treatment.[6] In 500 BC, Hippocrates described sciatica[6,7(p 753)], defined sciatica as *"radicular gluteal and posterior leg pain usually caused by impingement nerve roots at the L4-S1 root levels."* Galen and Aretaeus wrote of pain in the musculoskeletal and

Ithaca College Physician Assistant Program, Smiddy Hall 328, 953 Danby Road, Ithaca, NY 14850, USA
E-mail address: ssalahshor@ithaca.edu

Physician Assist Clin 9 (2024) 33–45
https://doi.org/10.1016/j.cpha.2023.08.002
2405-7991/24/© 2023 Elsevier Inc. All rights reserved.

nervous systems in 150 BC.[6] Centuries later, in the 1600sto 1800s, the description of back pain was attributed to rheumatological conditions.[6] The language, transcriptions, and written clinical cases about back pain continued to evolve.

The rheumatological system became the reason for LBP, at which time it was considered an illness without a cure.[8] According to Driscoll and colleagues,[9(p 976)] the anatomic definition of the lower back is *"the area on the poster aspect of the body from the lower margin of the twelfth ribs to the lower gluteal folds."* In the nineteenth century, back pain became known as a musculoskeletal system condition.[10] Today, like back then, clinicians grapple with the definition, diagnosis, and treatment of back pain due to the chronicity of its course and the biopsychosocial approach (**Fig. 1**) to manage back pain.[8,11] LBP frustrates clinicians and continues to be a complex and difficult presenting complaint to diagnose from top to bottom, and the differential list is extensive (**Table 1**).

BACKGROUND

LBP affects almost 90% of the global population at some point in their lifetime.[3,4,10,17] It remains the number one or two most common cause of musculoskeletal pain.[8] The global burden has a significant impact on the quality of life of the population affected, including physical pain, loss of work, loss of income, lack of function, and disability.[3,4,8,10,17] Back pain and its impact on daily life are overwhelming and challenging.

The International Association for the Study of Pain[12(p 1)] revised its definition of pain to *"an unpleasant sensory and emotional experience associated with or resembling that associated actual or potential tissue damage."* With the impact on the population overall, the approach to back pain is constantly changing. Clinicians use a biopsychosocial approach to evaluate back pain and arrive at a differential diagnosis. Biopsychosocial requires clinicians to look at anatomy, physiology, history, and physical, social, and emotional factors that contribute to LBP.[8] Clinicians across the globe agree that LBP is difficult to diagnose and manage.[17] With a new definition of pain, the multifactorial biopsychosocial approach, and the confounding factors, clinicians have their work cutout for them.

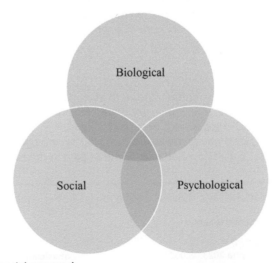

Fig. 1. Biopsychosocial approach.

Table 1
Definitions associated with back pain

Name	Definition
Pain	*"An unpleasant sensory and emotional experience associated with, or resembling that associated actual or potential tissue damage."*[12]
Low back pain/back pain	Posterior pain in the area at the lower margin of the 12th ribs to the lower gluteal folds with or without pain referred to one or both lower limbs.[13]
Acute back pain	Pain in the back for <28 d.[14]
Subacute back pain	Pain in the back for 28 d to 12 wk.[14]
Chronic back pain	Pain in the back for >120 d.[14]
Nonspecific back pain	Pain with no precise anatomic cause.[15]
Midline back pain	Back pain over the spinous processes.[7]
Paraspinal back pain	Back pain along and around the spinous processes.[7]
Sciatica	LBP, radiating down into L5 and S1 with paresthesia and weakness.[7]
Biopsychosocial approach	An approach that considers the clinical presentation of a patient, their work and activity, and their social and emotional factors.[8,16]

The Global Burden of Disease 2019 study recognized the challenge in clinicians' abilities to evaluate LBP. Patients present with LBP across their lifespan, as early as 5 years of age and beyond 90 years of age. In this context, LBP[3(p 2028)] is *"activity-limiting low back pain (± pain referred into 1 or both lower limbs) that last for at least 1 day."* Adults have a point prevalence of LBP between 12% and 33%, with a 1-year prevalence of 22% to 65%.[3] Adolescents' lifetime prevalence rate ranged from 7% to 72% with an adolescent experiencing LBP within the last year from 7% to 51%.[18] The elderly population (age > 65 years) prevalence was approximately 20%.[13] LBP affects all ages and is perplexing to arrive at a definite diagnosis.

The 1-year incidence spans a wide range from 2% to 40%.[17] The greatest incidence is in patients who are in their 30s.[3] The prevalence continues through to age 65 years when it begins to decline in incidence.[3] Across the ages, LBP limits the range of motion (ROM) which in turn limits activity and impacts other areas of patients' lives.[18,19] The burden on patients and families is real and has an impact beyond physical pain.

People who experience LBP limit their physical activity.[17] Recurrent LBP further adds burden for adults with the loss of productivity at work which leads to economic consequences.[17] LBP is the leading cause of disability across the world.[3,15] The Global Burden of Disease ranks LBP in the top 10 of diseases and injuries for disability.[15] Disability has a significant impact on the quality of life of patients.

The Global Burden of Disease 2019 study examined almost 400 diseases and injuries in more than 200 countries and territories.[20] The 2019 study reported the years lived with disability (YLDs) and disability-adjusted life years (DALYs). The addition of years of life lost and YLD equals DALYs.[21] Patients do not die from LBP; therefore, DALYs and YLDs are the same for LBP. To evaluate DALYs, measure the disability weight (DW) which looks at the severity of disease and injuries and ranges in value from 0 to 1.[21,22] The DW of acute and severe LBP with and without leg pain ranges from 0.269 to 0.374.[21,22] Therefore, early diagnosis and management of LBP directly impacts patients' daily activities.

In addition to the indirect cost associated with disability and time lost at work, there is a direct cost related to medical care.[4,14] The United States spends more than $100 billion on the indirect and direct costs associated with LBP.[4,14] Direct cost includes primary care visits and diagnostic tools used to evaluate and diagnose the etiology of LBP.

Undiagnosed nonspecific LBP leads to recurrence and chronic LBP. The burden of chronic back pain is even more costly, with the biggest impact on the ability to work and repeated visits to seek medical care.[2] The economic burden of chronic pain is in the billions of dollars for the United States.[2] Therefore, appropriate and timely diagnosis and management of back pain can decrease costs in the health care system.

Developing Differential Diagnoses

Physician Assistant/Associate are one of the primary care clinicians who are the first line for patients with acute, subacute, recurrent, and chronic LBP. Almost 10% of primary care clinicians must consider a broad range of diagnoses when evaluating patients with back pain.[23] Clinicians must evaluate LBP using the biopsychosocial approach and consider the risk factors. Risk factors are found in musculoskeletal and neurologic systems, such as degenerative disease, disruptions, cysts, birth defects, spondylosis, and spondylolisthesis.[24] Patients can have risk factors due to age, birth defects, high weight at the time of birth, gender, family history, history of surgery on the back or spine, and history of pregnancy.[24–26] These risk factors are beyond the control of patients.

Other risk factors include body weight, posture, physical activity lifestyle, mental health illnesses and conditions, type of occupation, sports activities, and chronic medical conditions.[24,25] The risk factors gathered from past medical, surgery, and social histories aid in the arrival of a differential diagnosis. A thorough and focused history is one key component to arriving at a differential diagnosis for lower back pain.

When taking a pain history, the Precipitating/Relieving, Quality, Region/Radiation, Severity scale, Timing (PQRST) pain assessment tool is often used (**Box 1**).[27,28] The PQRST pain assessment tool is used to ask historical questions using the prompts found in **Table 2**. Questions focus on the onset of pain, the location of pain, the characteristics of the pain, the duration of the pain, the severity of the pain, quantification using the pain scale, what makes the pain better or worse, does the pain radiate to anywhere else, the impact of an activity on pain, associated symptoms, the impact of the pain on activities of daily living, social activities, sleep, what medications help the pain, and whether pain is new, recurring, or chronic.[7,29,30]

A thorough history that includes the PQRST pain assessment tool will help produce an appropriate differential diagnosis. The onset of the pain categorizes the pain into acute, recurrent, or chronic. Location and radiation provide information about possible

---

Box 1
PQRST pain assessment

PQRST Pain Assessment Tool

P, Precipitating and Palliation

Q, Quality

R, Region/Radiation

S, Site and Severity scale

T, Timing

Adapted from: Swartz MH. The musculoskeletal system. In: Textbook of Physical Diagnosis History and Examination. 7th edition. Elsevier Saunders; 2014; page 519, Figure 1.

Table 2
History taking prompts

History Prompts	Type of Questions to Ask	Notes/Comments
Onset	When did the pain start? What were you doing when the pain started?	Today, yesterday, or last week
Location	*Point* to where the pain is?	L-spine region, S-spine region, midline of spine, along the lateral aspects of the spine
Characteristics (quality)	How does the pain feel? Is it constant or intermittent?	Dull, aching, throbbing, or sharp
Severity	On a scale of 1–10, how is the pain, 1 being not so bad but there, 10 being the worse pain ever?	
Factors that affect pain	What makes the pain better? What makes the pain worse?	Better: rest, medications Worse: movement, sitting, or standing
Radiation	Does the pain move anywhere else?	One leg, both legs, around the abdomen?
Impact of activity on pain	Does the pain limit your ability to work? Exercise? Take care of yourself or someone?	
Associated symptoms	Do you have any other symptoms?	Such as fever, nausea, vomiting, numbness, weakness in a limb, urinary incontinence, recent surgery, recent trauma
Impact of the pain on activities of daily living, social activities, and sleep	Are you able to do things that you like? Are you able to meet expectations of work, school, and family? Are you losing sleep because of the pain?	Psychosocial issues
New, recurring, or chronic	Is this the first time you have had this pain? Have you ever had this pain before, if so, when? Is this an ongoing pain, if so, what was the previous diagnosis and management?	Self-explanatory

causes of LBP. A thorough history also allows the clinician to evaluate for red flags that require immediate referral and help to rule out life-threatening diseases.[8,30]

During the history, inquire about numbness, incontinence, paresthesia, fever, trauma, weight loss, bleeding, pain at night, poor appetite, new LBP in adults 50 and older, no improvement after typical management for acute back pain, and history of cancer.[8] These symptoms can signal fracture, infection, cancer, or cauda equina syndrome.[8,19] An immediate referral is required for cauda equina syndrome, where the patient presents with urinary and neurologic symptoms.[8,15,19,29] A thorough history is essential to eliminate the serious causes of LBP. Red flag symptoms will need hospitalization and/or referral to a specialist.

The history must include questions to evaluate for yellow flags. **Table 3** has a list of yellow flags which are prognostic in nature and indicate biopsychological factors.[16,24,30] Recognizing the yellow flags related to work activities, personal beliefs, behaviors about the cause and management of LBP, and mental health illnesses, and conditions helps to develop a care plan that is comprehensive and patient-centered.[24,31]

After the history, the next step is the physical examination. Patient history guides the direction of the physical examination. The physical examination begins from the time the clinician enters the examination room. During that time, observe the patient's general appearance, body position, facial expression, and ability to move from the chair to the examination table.[7] The musculoskeletal examination includes inspection, palpation, joint movement or ROM, and specific techniques to assess the pain, labeled "IPROMS" ("I promise").[7,32] The neurologic examination includes the evaluation of L2, L3, L4, L5, and S1.[7,19,24,32] The physical examination helps narrow the differential diagnosis of the LBP.

The physical examination should occur with the patient in a gown for privacy and comfort while allowing full visualization of the back from cervical to sacral spine.[7] Inspection includes looking for masses, asymmetrical deformities, muscle wasting, erythema, and swelling.[7,32] Inspection should occur with the patient standing and walking in the examination room.[29] Inspecting gait should include the patient walking away from and toward the PA.[32] Gait is part of the inspection of the musculoskeletal physical examination.

Palpation follows inspection during the physical examination.[32] Palpation must include the entire spinous process and along the spine while talking to the patient.[24] Talking to the patient while examining them will give a better assessment of the severity of the pain.[7] The palpation of the spine should start away from the location of the pain.[29] Also consider the dermatome affected by the pain during palpation.[29] After inspection and palpation, the physician assistant/associate (PA) performs the ROM assessment.

The ROM of the lumbar spine includes flexion, extension, lateral bending, and rotation.[32] Lateral bending and rotation occur on both sides of the body.[30] Each movement has normal ranges and should be assessed.[32] Normal ROM for lumbar flexion is 75°, extension is 30°, lateral bending is 35°, and rotation is 30°.[32] After the history is obtained, red flags eliminated, yellow flags acknowledged and documented, the physical examination completed, and the differential diagnosis list is further prioritized.

The differential diagnoses for LBP are extensive. The structural, neurogenic, and extraspinal categories are used to differentiate the etiologies of LBP in **Box 2**.[23] Similar to this method is intrinsic versus systemic versus referred etiologies.[19] The location can be used to differentiate the cause of the LBP, along the spine versus on the spine.[7] Another method to differentiate the expansive etiology of LBP is based on specific conditions and their presentation.[29] Regardless of the process used to arrive at a differential, the gold standard is a thorough focus on history and physical examination.

Table 3
Yellow flags

Work Activities	Personal Beliefs	Behaviors	Mental Health Illnesses and Conditions
Cannot work until pain resolved	Assumes back pain is due to a serious condition, such as a fracture or cancer	Not engaged in the processes of getting better through therapies such as physical therapy	Depression
Afraid to work due to fear pain will return or get worse	Wrongly labels signs and symptoms experienced	Stop engagement in social events that include exertion	Anxiety
History of not working consistently	In denial about the possibility that LBP will resolve	Poor sleep habits due to pain	Partner is too involved or not involved
The work environment is not ergonomically focused	Not a person who likes to do physical activity if recommended	Use of alcohol or other substance to cope with the pain	Support system nonexisting

---

Box 2
Outline differential diagnosis of low back pain

I. Structural etiologies of low back pain
  1. Lumbar intervertebral discs
     a. High-intensity zones and annular tears
     b. Degenerative disc disease
     c. Diskitis
  2. Zygapophysial joints and capsules
     a. Facet joint degeneration
     b. Facet hypertrophy
     c. Capsular derangement and calcification
  3. Sacroiliac joint
     a. SI joint arthropathy
     b. SI joint instability
  4. Ligamentum flavum
  5. Dura mater and arachnoid structures
  6. Pelvic insufficiency fracture
  7. Vertebral bodies
     a. Vertebral fractures
     b. Spondylolysis, spondylolisthesis, and pars defects
  8. Musculoligamentous structure
     a. Paralumbar muscular conditions
     b. Spinal ligament derangement
     c. Instability of the lumbar structure
     d. Piriformis syndrome
     e. Myofascial etiology
  9. Iatrogenic etiologies
     a. Instrumentation
     b. Lumbar surgery

II. Neurogenic etiologies of low back Pain
  1. Spinal stenosis
     a. Central and foraminal spinal stenosis (degenerative)
        i. Degenerative disc disease
        ii. Facet hypertrophy and arthropathy
        iii. Ligamentum flavum hypertrophy
        iv. Vertebral fractures
        v. Neoplastic
        vi. Abscess formation
        vii. Hematoma formation
        viii. Iatrogenic because of leaked vetebro or kyphoplasty residue
     b. Congenital and developmental
        i. Incomplete vertebral arch closure
        ii. Segmentation failure
        iii. Achondroplasia
        iv. Shortened pedicles
        v. Spina bifida
        vi. Thoracolumbar kyphosis
        vii. Apical vertebral wedging
        viii. Osseous exostosis

III. Extraspinal etiologies of low back pain
  1. Rheumatologic conditions
  2. Gastrointestinal
  3. Pelvic and gynecologic
  4. Vascular
  5. Infection
  6. Neoplasms
  7. Psychological

Abbreviation: SI, sacroiliac.

From Swartz MH. The musculoskeletal system. In: *Textbook of Physical Diagnosis History and Examination* .7th edition. Elsevier Saunders; 2014; page 519, Figure 1.

The onset of LBP guides the differential diagnosis. *Is it acute? It is chronic? Did it start and gradually progress?* The most common cause of LBP has no identifiable cause, known as nonspecific back pain.[15] **Fig. 2** shows the causes of acute LBP associated with a traumatic injury.[8] Based on the history, physical examination, and appropriate musculoskeletal and neurologic assessments, the cause of the acute LBP due to traumatic injury can be diagnosed.[8] Meanwhile, nonspecific LBP can present a frustrating challenge. The use of a methodical process of eliminating differential causes is a guidepost to alleviate the frustration.

The structural versus neurologic versus extraspinal method has an extensive list of etiologies to consider. Intervertebral disc tears, bulges, herniations, tears, and in some cases, infections due to surgical procedures are structural causes.[23] Internal disc disruption (IDD) is seen in adolescents to middle-aged patients.[26] Approximately 30% to 35% of structural causes of LBP emanate from the facet joint.[23,26] Sacroiliac joint pain accounts for about 20% of structural LBP.[23,26] Although IDD, facet joint pain, and sacroiliac joint pain are the most common causes of structural causes of LBP, there are others worth mentioning.

There can also be LBP from inflammation of the dura mater and arachnoid structures.[23] LBP due to an inflammatory process is typically gradual in onset.[33] Ankylosing spondylitis is an example of an inflammatory condition with presenting back pain. Past medical history is essential in identifying inflammatory causes of LBP.[8,33] Fractures of

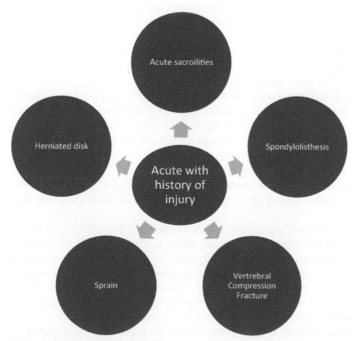

Fig. 2. Causes of acute low back pain (LBP).

the vertebral body also fall into the structural categories as well as pelvic insufficiency fractures and musculoligamentous conditions. Patients with vertebral body fractures may have a history of osteoporosis, a history of steroid use, or be more than 60 years of age.[34] With so many differential diagnoses to consider in patients who present with LBP, the skill of taking a thorough past medical history is the key to arriving at an appropriate differential diagnosis.

Performing the history, physical examination, and assessment of which physical examination diagnostic tool to use to determine structural versus neurogenic causes of LBP require skills. Developing a viable differential diagnosis of LBP due to structural versus neurogenic also poses a challenge due to the overlap.[23] Spinal stenosis, a neurogenic cause of LBP, is decreased volume in the spinal canal.[35] Lumbar spinal stenosis should be considered when an older patient presents with LBP and the pain is unchanged with ambulation and worse with activities such as sitting down.[35] Patients with spinal stenosis present with complaints that suggest radicular and neurogenic pain due to nerve root compression.[8] Another neurogenic cause of back pain that requires discussion is degenerative disc disease. Patients present with pain in the neck and back.[36] The history questions that ask about what makes the pain worse or better help in narrowing the differential diagnosis to include degenerative disc disease.[36] Fractures, cancer, abscess, hematomas, and iatrogenic causes of LBP differentiation are more likely to be considered based on the history and confirmed with the physical examination and other diagnostic tools. The history will also differentiate congenital and developmental causes (see **Box 1**) by presentation at birth, such as incomplete vertebral arch closure and spina bifida, by routine evaluation of milestone development, segmentation failure, and achondroplasia.

The physical examination should include specific tests performed during the musculoskeletal and neurologic examination. Lasegue's test is commonly known as the straight leg raise test. The straight leg test is positive if, during the physical examination, the patient has pain with flexion of the hip and extension of the knee.[7,8] There is also Bragard's sign where the additional dorsiflexion of the foot elicits pain during the straight leg test.[8] A positive Lasegue's test and Bragard's sign on physical examination maneuvers suggest pain LBP due to a radiculopathy condition such as compression fractures and cancer.[7,8]

LBP can be due to pain outside of the spine—extraspinal or referred pain.[19,23,37] An abdominal aortic aneurysm is a cardiac cause of LBP, and the patient presents with a history of abdominal, flank, and back pain, with a pulsatile abdominal mass on abdominal physical examination.[8,19,23,33] Herpes zoster is another extraspinal etiology where patients present with LBP and a rash distribution following a dermatome.[19,38] If there is a rash, inquire about a history of chickenpox.[38] With such an extensive differential diagnosis list in patients who present with LBP, the skills of getting the history and performing a physical examination that is thorough will determine the next steps for patients.

Although the history and physical examination are the essence of the evaluation of LBP, there are indications for imaging studies. The literature does not recommend routine imaging such as MRI and computed tomography (CT) in patients who present with LBP.[19,34,39] A thorough history and focused and comprehensive physical examination determine the need for imaging. Red flag etiologies require imaging and the referred specialist will determine the appropriate imaging.[39] Extraspinal or referred causes of LBP require laboratory testing, including a complete blood count with differential, erythrocyte sedimentation rate, metabolic panel, and urinalysis if an inflammatory, infectious, or malignant cause is part of the differential diagnosis.[19,24] Clinicians can order laboratory and imaging studies based on their differential diagnosis at the time of referral.

SUMMARY

Primary care PAs see acute, recurrent, and chronic LBP every day in their practice. The history, physical examination, and use of special physical examination techniques are critical in determining the laboratory and diagnostic tools to use to arrive at a differential diagnosis and manage the LBP of patients. The thorough, focused, and comprehensive history informs the physical examination done, determines the imaging needed, and narrows the differential diagnoses considered. Narrowing the differential diagnoses leads to the appropriate intervention and referral. Early and focused intervention helps to avoid and/or limit disability and avoid increased pain and chronicity of LBP.

CLINICS CARE POINTS

- The history and physical examination remain the gold standard to arrive at an appropriate differential diagnosis of low back pain (LBP).
- Rule out the presence of red flags with LBP and refer immediately if present.
- Consider the yellow flags in the patient who presents with LBP due to their impact on outcomes.
- Do not routinely order laboratory and diagnostic tools in the assessment of LBP.
- Treatment is specific to the condition or illness causing the symptom of LBP.

DISCLOSURE

No disclosure.

REFERENCES

1. Hoy D, March L, Brooks P, et al. Measuring the global burden of low back pain. Best Pract Res Clin Rheumatol 2010;24(2):155–65.
2. Gore M, Sadosky BP, Tai KS, et al. The burden of chronic low back pain. Spine 2012;37(11):E668–77.
3. Hoy D, Bain C, Williams G, et al. A systematic review of the global prevalence of low back pain. Arthritis Rheum 2012;64(6):2028–37.
4. Buchbinder R, Blyth FM, March LM, et al. Placing the global burden of low back pain in context. Best Pract Res Clin Rheumatol 2013;27(5):575–89.
5. Lucas JW, Connor EM, Bose J. Back, lower limb pain among U.S. adults, 2019. NCHS Data Brief, no 415. Hyattsville, MD. National Center for Health Statistics 2021;107894. https://doi.org/10.15620/cdc.
6. Allan DB, Waddell G. An historical perspective on low back pain and disability. Acta Orthopaedica Scandinavia 1989;60(sup234):1–23.
7. Bickley LS, Szilagyi PG, Hoffman RM. Musculoskeletal system. In: Bickley LS, editor. Bates' Guide to Physical Examination and History Taking. 13th ed. Philadelphia, PA: Wolters Kluwer; 2021. p. 745–840.
8. Gibbs D, McGahan BG, Ropper AE, et al. Back pain: differential diagnosis and management. Neuro Clin 2023;41(1):1–23.

9. Driscoll T, Jacklyn G, Orchard J, et al. The global burden of occupationally related low back pain: estimates from the Global Burden of Disease 2010 study. Ann Rheum Dis 2014;73(6):2630–7.

10. Hoy D, March L, Brooks, et al. The global burden of low back pain: estimates from the Global Burden of Disease 2010 study. Ann Rheum Dis 2014;73(6):968–74.

11. Buchbinder R, van Tulder M, Oberg B, et al, Lancet Low Back Pain Series Working Group. Low back pain: a call for action. Lancet 2018;391(6):2384–8.

12. The International Association for the Study of Pain. IASP announces revised definition of pain. International Association for the Study of Pain (IASP). Published July 16, 2020. https://www.iasp-pain.org/publications/iasp-news/iasp-announces-revised-definition-of-pain/. Accessed April 16, 2023.

13. Dionne CE, Dunn KM, Croft PR. Does back pain prevalence really decrease with increasing age? A systematic review. Age Ageing 2006;35(3):229–34.

14. Qaseem A, Wilt TJ, Mclean RM, et al. Noninvasive treatments for acute, subacute, and chronic low back pain: a clinical practice guideline from the American College of Physicians. Ann Intern Med 2017;166(7):514–30.

15. Maher C, Underwood M, Buchbinder R. Non-specific low back pain. Lancet 2017;389(10070):736–47.

16. Keeley P, Creed F, Tomenson B, et al. Psychosocial predictors of health-related quality of lifeand health service utilisation in people with chronic low back pain. Paint 2008;135(1):142–50.

17. Hoy D, Brooks P, Blyth F, et al. The epidemiology of low back pain. Best Pract Res Clin Rheumatol 2010;24(6):769–81.

18. Jeffries LJ, Milanese SF, Grimmer-Somers KA. Epidemiology of adolescent spinal pain: a systematic overview of the research literature. Spine 2007;32(23):2630–7.

19. Casazza BA. Diagnosis and treatment of acute low back pain. Am Fam Physician 2012;85(4):343–50. https://www.aafp.org/pubs/afp/issues/2012/0215/p343.html?utm_medium=referral&utm_source=r360.

20. Vos T, Lim SS, Abbafati C, et al. Global burden of 369 diseases and injuries in 204 countries and territories, 1990-2019: a systematic analysis for the Global Burden of Disease Study 2019. Lancet 2020;396(10258):1204–22.

21. Murray CJL. Quantifying the burden of disease: the technical basis for disability-adjusted life years. Bull World Health Organ 1994;72(3):429–45.

22. Charalampous P, Polinder S, Wothge J, et al. A systematic literature review of disability weights measurement studies: evolution of methodological choices. Arch Public Health 2022;80:91.

23. Amirdelfan K, McRoberts P, Deer TR. The differential diagnosis of low back pain: a primer on the evolving paradigm. Neuromodulation 2014;17(3):209–13.

24. Webb CW, O'Connor FG. Low back pain in primary care: an evidence-based approach. In: South-Paul JE, Matheny SC, Lewis EL, editors. Current Diagnosis & Treatment: Family Medicine. 4th ed. New York, NY: McGraw Hill Education; 2015. p. 250–60.

25. Krasin E, Schermann H, Snir N, et al. A quick guide and comprehensive guide to the differential diagnosis of neck and back pain: a narrative review. SN Comp Clin Med 2022;4(1):1–9.

26. DePalma MJ, Ketchum JM, Saulio T. What is the source of chronic low back pain and does age play a role? Pain Med 2011;12(2):224–33.

27. Pain Assessment: Practice essentials, overview, technique. eMedicine. Published online October 26, 2022. https://emedicine.medscape.com/article/1948069-overview?icd=login_success_email_match_norm#showall. Accessed March 3, 2023.

28. Gauchan S. Pain assessment in the emergency department of a teaching hospital in Lalitpur. Journal of Karnali Academy of Health Sciences 2019;2(3):209–13.
29. Chatterjee R. Low back pain assessment: the 10 minute consultation. Co-Kinetic Journal 2016;70:18–25. Accessed February 1, 2023.
30. Jensen S. Back pain-clinical assessment. Aust Fam Physician 2004;33(6):393–401. https://search.informit.org/doi/10.3316/informit.373076018335835.
31. Henschke N, Maher CG, Refshauge KM, et al. Characteristics of patients with acute low back pain presenting to the primary care in Australia. Clin J Pain 2009;25(1):11.
32. Swartz MH. The musculoskeletal system. In: Swartz MH, editor. Textbook of Physical Diagnosis History and Examination. 7th edition. Philadelphia, PA: Elsevier/Saunders; 2014. p. 533–82.
33. Filatova ES, ShF Erdes, Filatova EG. Differential diagnosis of inflammatory and mechanical back pain. J Neurol Psychol 2016;116(6):104–8.
34. Chou R, Qaseem A, Snow V, et al. Diagnosis and treatment of low back pain: a joint clinical practice guideline from the American College of Physicians and the American Pain Society. Ann Int Med 2007;147(7):478–91.
35. Kriener DS, Shaffer WO, Baiseden JL, et al. An evidence-based clinical guideline for the diagnosis and treatment of degenerative lumbar spinal stenosis (update). Spine J 2013;13(7):734–43.
36. Tonosu J, Inanami H, Oka H, et al. Diagnosing discogenic low back pain associated with degenerative disc disease using a medical interview. PLoS One 2016;11(11):e0166031.
37. Thalmann NF, Rimensberger C, Blum MR, et al. Internist differential diagnosis in acute back pain. Journ Rheum 2023;82(1):13–8.
38. Kelley A. Herpes Zoster: a primary care approach to diagnosis and treatment. JAAPA 2022;35(12):13–8.
39. Oliveira CB, Maher CG, Pinto RZ, et al. Clinical practice guidelines for the management of non-specific low back pain in primary care: an updated overview. Euro Spine Journ 2018;27(11):2791–803.

Hip Pain: What Could it Mean?

Amie D. Beals, PA-C

KEYWORDS

- Hip pain • Greater trochanteric pain syndrome • Hip osteoarthritis
- Femoroacetabular impingement • Avascular necrosis of the hip
- Lumbar nerve impingement • Hip labral injury • Hip fracture

KEY POINTS

- The skill of taking a history regarding hip pain is integral to obtaining the information necessary to make an accurate diagnosis, a timely referral, and a definitive treatment plan.
- Hip pain affects 12% to 40% of adults greater than 50 years of age on a daily basis.
- Common pathology for hip pain, including greater trochanteric pain syndrome, osteoarthritis, femoroacetabular impingement, avascular necrosis, labral injury, hip fracture, lumbar nerve impingement, and septic arthritis, is elucidated by asking appropriate historical questions in a logical manner.

INTRODUCTION

Adult hip pain can be an annoyance as simple as everyday activities getting interrupted to take a mild pain reliever, or it can be a debilitating condition that rules every minute of every day. As practitioners, we have been charged with the responsibility of getting to the root of the problem in a timely manner with as little waste of resources as possible. The skill of taking a history regarding hip pain is integral to beginning this process and leads to appropriate testing, a more accurate diagnosis, a timely referral, and a definitive treatment to aid in the relief of symptoms. Several studies have reported that in patients older than 50 years of age, the prevalence of hip pain ranges from 12% to 40%,[1,2] which is a staggering number of patients who live with this condition on a daily basis. By asking the right questions, and carefully listening to the answers of our patients, the challenge to diagnose and treat common sources of hip pain is greatly decreased. In this article, the art of the practitioner-patient interview leading to the correct cause of adult hip pain is outlined.

DISCUSSION

As clinicians working in family practice, urgent care, emergency medicine, general surgery, orthopedics, or a multitude of other areas of medicine, having the ability to significantly narrow down an adult patient's complaint of hip pain is essential; however, it is

Springfield Orthopaedics and Sports Medicine Institute, 140 West Main Street, Suite 100, Springfield, OH 45502, USA
E-mail address: adbealspac@gmail.com

Physician Assist Clin 9 (2024) 47–58
https://doi.org/10.1016/j.cpha.2023.07.007
2405-7991/24/© 2023 Elsevier Inc. All rights reserved.
physicianassistant.theclinics.com

nearly impossible without the masterful skill of listening and taking a thorough history. According to some studies, patients with intra-articular hip pathology see an average of 3.3 clinicians before a clear diagnosis is established.[3,4] Thus, an informed, systematic approach to assessment and diagnosis is important. This approach can lead to much more definitive answers when investigating an unknown pathologic condition of the hip and directs the examination, testing, diagnosis, and possible referral, and leads to quicker treatment. Of course, history alone cannot render a diagnosis, but it certainly narrows the focus.

Two separate studies, over 4 and 6 weeks, respectively, reported that 11.99% of adults older than age 65 in Italy, and 14.3% older than age 60 in the United States experienced hip pain on most days.[1,2] In a larger study, among adults who play sports, the incidence of chronic hip pain is 30% to 40%.[5,6] This showcases that hip pain is a significant problem in the adult population. Hip pain can range from a minor irritation limiting sporting activities or grocery shopping to a debilitating condition affecting every aspect of life and can have many different causes.

The method used to elicit useful information leading to a definitive diagnosis should be modified according to the patient's ability to converse and to describe signs and symptoms of their hip pain. The ability to focus on each patient's individual story then leads to a more concise examination. This saves time and money and allows the clinician to focus on the patient's primary concern initiating the visit.

METHODS

The questions a practitioner asks, and the order in which they are presented, can significantly affect the duration of a visit and the confidence a patient has in the practitioner's ability to determine the solution to their hip pain. Starting with a clear statement, such as, "I see that you've been scheduled to be evaluated for hip pain today," notifies the patient that the clinician is aware of the specific problem and is interested in discovering more about that particular issue. It also focuses the patient on the hip and avoids veering into other conversations. As the discussion develops, many other questions then follow regarding the quality, timing, and exacerbating factors of their hip pain. The line of questioning should logically follow an "if this, then that," or algorithmic, approach that leads to the answers the clinician needs to solve the mystery of the source of the hip pain. Several algorithmic approaches have been described in the literature according to the location of pain,[7,8] a structural layer approach,[9] and an intra-articular versus extra-articular approach.[10] Because these approaches all have validation in the clinical arena, no single algorithmic approach applies to every patient. Flexibility in the line of questioning and tailoring the inquiry to each patient is essential.

Encouraging patients to explain how their symptoms are affecting them in their everyday life is an appropriate place to start their hip pain narrative. A patient typically presents for evaluation when it is keeping them awake at night, affecting their ability to navigate stairs to get to their bathroom or bedroom, keeping them from being able to walk distances or stand for long periods of time, or limiting participation in their exercise program or extracurricular activities. Some explain how it keeps them from performing their job, which leads to days off work thereby affecting their income. Knowing their motivation to seek care and return to more normal activities is important in directing a treatment program.

Greater Trochanteric Pain Syndrome

If a patient's pain is keeping them awake at night, follow that with a line of questioning regarding why it keeps them awake. Is the pain positional, such as when they lie on one side or the other? Greater trochanteric pain syndrome (GTPS) (formerly known as trochanteric bursitis) is one of the most common findings in patients with this complaint. The best estimates of prevalence demonstrated unilateral GTPS was present in 15% of women and 6.6% of men in a large, community-based study with more than 3000 adults aged 50 to 70 years.[11] The female-to-male ratio is approximately 4:1 and the usual age at presentation is older than 50 years.[11]

Another question to narrow the diagnosis to GTPS is to ask, "Has your gait changed for any reason lately?" Overuse of the hip and a change in the way a person walks (or a limp) are common contributing factors in developing GTPS, therefore patients with this condition have a positive response to this question much of the time. If direct palpation of the area of pain elicits tenderness over the lateral area of the greater trochanter, this is indicative of the condition. This physical finding coupled with a normal hip radiograph further narrows the diagnosis. Nonsteroidal anti-inflammatory medications (NSAIDs), stretching, physical therapy, corticosteroid injection over the area of the greater trochanteric bursa, and correcting the abnormal gait are all viable therapeutic options for GTPS. If these modalities do not improve the symptoms, referral to an orthopedic specialist is recommended.

Osteoarthritis

If the pain is keeping them awake at night, but it is described as a constant dull aching located more in the groin or buttock, the findings are more likely consistent with an intra-articular condition, such as arthritis (osteo, psoriatic, or rheumatoid) or avascular necrosis (AVN) of the hip. Next, asking the patient, "Does it also bother you during the day?" provides the clinician with greater context. Morning stiffness, or stiffness after sitting for an extended period of time (ie, when eating at a restaurant or going to a movie), and increased pain in the groin or buttock with extended periods of walking or standing, also indicate that the location of the pain is centered in the hip joint itself. On examination, limited range of motion and pain with passive internal rotation of the hip are most common with osteoarthritis and significantly narrow the focus of the patient's pain generator. In those with very advanced osteoarthritis, the patient may also have limited external rotation of the hip, at which time the patient complains of difficulty in being able to lift the foot to don socks and shoes. Referred pain to the knee is another common complaint of patients with hip osteoarthritis.

The hip is the third most common joint affected by osteoarthritis after the knee and the hand[12] and women are affected more than men. In adults older than 45 years, 6.7% to 9.7% will have osteoarthritis of the hip and one in four adults who live to age 85 will develop symptomatic hip osteoarthritis in their lifetime.[13,14] As patients age, the prevalence of hip osteoarthritis climbs with the highest incidence in the 60- to 64-year age category.[14] Plain film radiographs in at least two views, most commonly anterior-posterior (AP) and cross-table lateral or frog-leg view, are best for this diagnosis. Findings on radiograph positively identifying osteoarthritis include narrowing of the normal hip joint space of 2 to 2.5 mm,[15] sclerosis, bony cysts, and osteophytes. Combining the history, the physical findings, and the radiographic findings with a diagnostic and therapeutic intra-articular corticosteroid injection can confirm the diagnosis by relieving pain. Depending on the degree of pain the patient expresses, NSAIDs, assistive walking devices (eg, a cane or walker), and repeated corticosteroid injections are the mainstay of treatment until these modalities no longer provide pain relief; then referral to an orthopedist for discussion of definitive surgical intervention is indicated.

Femoroacetabular Impingement Syndrome

Femoroacetabular impingement (FAI) syndrome is caused by abnormal contact of the femoral head-neck junction and the acetabular rim causing anterior groin pain. In this regard, similar to osteoarthritis, FAI may elicit similar answers to questions regarding the location of hip pain. In contrast to osteoarthritis, hip impingement, as FAI is also called, does tend to occur more in males than females, and more often occurs in a younger population, with the average age between 20 and 45. It is also more common in athletes.[16] When asked to locate their pain, patients sometimes demonstrate it by putting the palm of the hand over the lateral hip area with the thumb pointing anteriorly and the fingers toward the buttock, thereby forming a "C" around the hip. This is effectively called the "C-sign" and can lead to more specific questions regarding FAI.

After observing the C-sign, "When is your pain most noticeable?" is an appropriate follow-up question because, in contrast to osteoarthritis, pain caused by FAI is most often noted after sitting with the hips flexed to 90° for extended periods of time, such as working at a desk, riding in a car or airplane, or sitting at the movies. As it progresses, athletic endeavors become more painful, as does navigating stairs. "What relieves your pain?" also produces a unique answer in that standing and walking tend to provide relief.

The confirmatory examination of a patient in whom the clinician suspects FAI would produce pain with the "impingement test," or flexion-adduction-internal rotation test, which involves bending the knee and hip to 90° and internally rotating the hip. Typically, hip radiographs demonstrate the cam lesion (bony lesion on the head/neck junction of the femur), pincer lesion (extra bone growth on the rim of the acetabulum), or both. Treatment of hip impingement may initially be conservative in nature with NSAIDs, rest, avoidance of painful activities, and intra-articular corticosteroid injections. If this is not successful in relieving pain, surgical intervention may be indicated; therefore, referral to an orthopedic surgeon may be necessary.

Avascular Necrosis (Osteonecrosis)

The line of questioning leading to a diagnosis of AVN, or osteonecrosis, can follow a similar path as osteoarthritis and FAI of the hip, and although pain is noted with range of motion, limitation of range of motion is typically not as common, and radiographic findings are different. AVN is more common in men than women and the age range at diagnosis is typically 35 to 50 years of age, with the average age of presentation being 44 years old.[17] The younger age at presentation, coupled with questions regarding possible risk factors, can lead the clinician to this diagnosis. Risk factors include extended use of glucocorticoids, excessive alcohol intake, smoking, systemic lupus erythematosus, posttransplant status, trauma to the hip, genetic disorders affecting blood flow (including sickle cell disease), HIV, radiation therapy, acute lymphoblastic leukemia,[18] and other less prominent risks.

Standard radiographs are not as definitive early in the course of the disease, but the "crescent sign" is appreciated as progression occurs. The crescent sign is a subchondral lucency seen most frequently in the anterolateral aspect of the proximal femoral head and is typically best appreciated in the lateral view. If AVN is suspected despite a negative hip radiograph, an MRI without contrast, with greater than 99% sensitivity and specificity,[19] is the imaging of choice to further delineate the severity and extent of involvement of the femoral head because vascular flow is compromised leading to collapse of the bone.

Referral to an orthopedic specialist is indicated to define the management and treatment options for a patient with this condition. If proven stable, AVN may be treated much like osteoarthritis of the hip with NSAIDs, walking aids, and intra-articular corticosteroid injections. When proven unstable, or when pain becomes uncontrollable with conservative measures, surgical intervention may be indicated with core decompression, bone grafting, and osteotomy. When these measures fail, demonstrated by lack of pain relief, or if the disease at the time of presentation is proven to be aggressive, or beyond the ability to preserve the femoral head (>30% of the head), a total hip arthroplasty may be indicated.[20]

Adult Exacerbation of Legg-Calve-Perthes and Slipped Capital Femoral Epiphysis

Knowing how long the pain has been present is also important. Ask the patient if the pain began years ago and has just now elevated to the point of affecting their activities of daily living, as in an arthritic hip, or were they playing pickleball last week and noted pain thereafter, as in a strain of hip tendons, or even a fracture? If the pain is long-standing and the location of the pain is in the groin, this may be osteoarthritis, but also ask questions regarding their childhood for possible findings consistent with Legg-Calve-Perthes or slipped capital femoral epiphysis. AVN caused by Legg-Calve-Perthes or slipped capital femoral epiphysis is the underlying diagnosis in approximately 10% of all total hip replacements in the United States.[18]

As a child, the patient may have had pain in the hip that improved with time or had surgery to stabilize the femoral head, but in adulthood, the pain has returned and a limp is noticed (because of pain itself, or because of shortening of the leg relative to the collapse of the femoral head). They may also describe one leg as being smaller than the other, possibly caused by atrophy of the thigh musculature. When asked about the motion that causes pain, the patient may complain of pain in the groin with flexion and/or abduction of the hip. A plain film AP view of the hip typically confirms this diagnosis with great accuracy. Again, orthopedic referral is advised to further discuss possible conservative versus surgical interventions to alleviate the pain (**Fig. 1**).

Soft Tissue Injury

Acute symptoms of hip pain after an injury or athletic event can also be a source of concern for normally active adult patients. During the interview, the patient may know the exact time the pain began, such as an athletic activity or during exercise. If the patient also describes a bulge in the groin, consider further evaluation for an inguinal hernia. Other sequential questions to further narrow the diagnosis are regarding the location of the pain, improvement or worsening of the pain since the time of injury, attempted home remedies (ice, NSAIDs, rest, stretching), and effect on their activities of daily living and sleep. Ligament and tendon injury symptoms are typically described as pain with certain movements of the hip requiring muscular contraction. Everyday activities, such as climbing the stairs (hip flexors anteriorly in the hip/groin include iliopsoas, sartorius, rectus femoris, tensor fasciae latae, and pectineus; hip extensors posteriorly in the buttocks are gluteus medius and maximus; quadriceps in the front of the thigh; and the hamstrings in the back of the thigh), getting in and out of the car (hip abductors and adductors, and iliotibial band), and squatting to sit on a chair or toilet (quadriceps, hamstrings, and glutes), can narrow the focus to certain muscle groups that may have been strained during the activity.

Typical treatment modalities for hip strains involve NSAIDs, ice, rest, rest, and more rest, and physical therapy. The patient usually admits to modest improvement of a soft tissue injury with these therapies over a relatively short period of time, but lingering mild symptoms can last anywhere up to 3 months, especially in hip flexor and hamstring strains. Hip radiographs typically have no acute or chronic abnormalities in a simple strain.

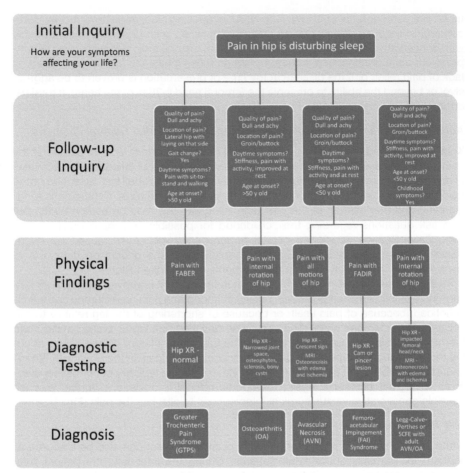

Fig. 1. Evaluation for hip pain during sleep. FABER, fexion-abduction-external rotation; FADIR, flexion-adduction-internal rotation; SCFE, slipped capital femoral epiphysis.

Labral Injury

Other acute hip injuries with anteriorly located pain can lead to the discovery of labral pathology. Rarely, labral tears can cause buttock pain, if the tear is located laterally or posteriorly. During the acute hip pain line of questioning, also ask, "Do you notice any painful catching, clicking, or locking of the hip?" Typically, nonpainful noises and clicking are of minimal significance, but when pain is associated with the sensation of catching or locking, a torn labrum may be the source. Labral tears are usually most painful with activity and rest provides relief of symptoms. Degenerative tears of the labrum, most common in the anterior and superior quadrants, which create the anteriorly located hip pain, are common and may be an incidental finding on a hip MRI or MRI arthrogram (most accurate testing for labral tears[21]). However, without mechanical symptoms, the labrum is not likely the source of the pain and may require no treatment. Physical testing of the hip induces pain in the extremes of range of motion and the flexion-adduction-internal rotation test is typically positive for pain when an anterior tear is present.[22] Hip radiographs may find hip dysplasia or may be normal. If mechanical symptoms are associated with pain, and MRI demonstrates a labral tear, referral to an orthopedist is indicated for further evaluation and treatment.

Femoral Neck and Pelvic Fracture

At any age, a history of an acute injury, such as a fall from a height or a car accident, is also a common cause of acute hip pain that may lead to the finding of an acute proximal femoral fracture or pelvic fracture. Acetabular and pubic rami fractures can produce groin pain that can last for 2 to 3 months. Stress fractures of the femoral neck may also occur in the setting of training overload during the patient's professional or athletic activities, such as dancers, endurance athletes, and military service members.[23] Again, the questions asked in the interview are critical in leading to the proper diagnosis, and asking about extracurricular activities is essential. A patient in the age range of 20 to 30 years of age who participates in these types of activities would alert the clinician to investigate further for a fracture. Insufficiency fractures because of compromised bone strength also occur without trauma in postmenopausal women.

If not recognized and treated, nondisplaced, stress, and insufficiency fractures can progress to complete and displaced fractures with high rates of nonunion and AVN. If the fracture is nondisplaced, it may not be visualized on initial injury radiographs, but answers to the clinician's questions regarding timing, persistence of pain, and relieving factors paint the picture of an acute fracture and thereby lead to more investigation.[24] Typically, an acute fracture, whether caused by an injury or the completion of a stress or insufficiency fracture, causes sudden pain in the groin and persistent pain with ambulation despite considerable conservative management with rest, pain medications, and weight-bearing restrictions. Physical examination often demonstrates pain with passive range of motion of the hip in all directions. Serial radiographs or MRI[25] can aid in diagnosis. Other acute injuries that can contribute to hip pain are not in the hip at all, but instead, have an origin in the back (**Fig. 2**).

Lumbar Spine and Sacroiliac Joint Pathology Causing Hip Pain

Differentiating hip pathology from spine or sacroiliac joint pathology also requires a critical line of questioning and investigation. It is estimated that up to 50% to 80% of adults have low back pain at some time in their lives.[26] If a patient complains of anterior hip pain or buttock pain, but the plain film radiograph is negative for obvious hip arthritis, FAI, or AVN pathology, and no injury history is noted, strongly consider further evaluation of the lumbar spine. Asking about the quality and character of the pain is integral in delineating hip versus back pain in many instances.

Open-ended questions, such as, "Tell me about how your pain feels. Is it sharp, aching, burning, constant, throbbing, shooting, cramping, or feel different in another way?" help the patient to describe their pain in terms that then lead the astute clinician down a narrower algorithmic pathway. Burning pain, or pain that has an "electric character" may be more suggestive of lumbar spine pathology, especially if accompanied by associated numbness or weakness.[27] Asking about a history of back pain or surgery is essential, and questions regarding the temporal and postural occurrence of the pain can further define its origin. Spinal stenosis, or narrowing of the spinal canal, rarely causes pain at rest, whereas, in contrast, standing erect for extended periods of time tends to cause the most pain.[28] The "shopping cart sign" is one of the hallmark historical reports from a patient with spinal stenosis, meaning that leaning over a shopping cart at the grocery relieves their pain.

Next ask, "Does the pain that you're having travel anywhere down the legs?" Impingement of the L3 nerve root causes pain in the distribution of the nerve innervating the area of the anterior groin and may cause weakness in the hip flexor and

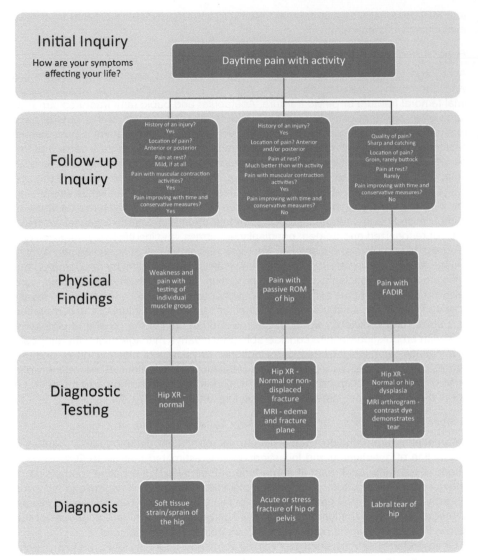

Fig. 2. Evaluation for hip pain during the day with activity. ROM, range of motion.

hip adductor musculature.[27] This is a common confounding and confusing symptom when teasing out the cause of hip pain. Sacroiliac origin of pain typically is located just lateral to the lumbar spine on one side or the other and is typically tender to palpation. Pain radiating down the posterior aspect of the leg is indicative of sciatic nerve involvement. Positive FABER (flexion-abduction-external rotation), compression, distraction, thigh thrust, and Gaenslen tests further identify the patient's pain generator to be located in the sacroiliac joint. Testing for lumbar nerve impingement pathology includes positive findings of weakness in one or both lower extremities, decreased deep tendon reflexes, decreased sensation, and positive straight-leg raise/crossed straight-leg raise and/or femoral stretch test/crossed femoral stretch test.[29]

Initial treatment with NSAIDs, oral steroids, physical therapy, muscle relaxers, medications for neuropathic pain (gabapentin or pregabalin), and epidural, sacroiliac joint,

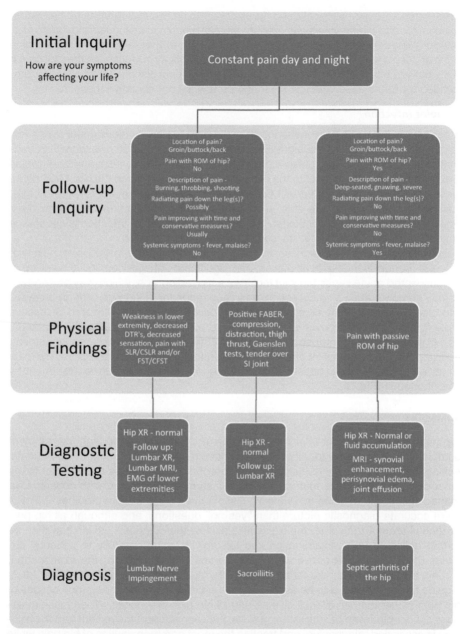

Fig. 3. Evaluation for constant hip pain during the day and night. CFST, crossed femoral stretch test; CSLR, crossed straight-leg raise; DTR, deep tendon reflex; EMG, electromyogram; FADIR, flexion-adduction-internal rotation; FST, femoral stretch test; SI, sacroiliac; SLR, straight-leg raise.

or facet corticosteroid injections may be helpful to treat the pain and to further narrow the diagnosis. The exception to this is in a rare instance of progressive lower extremity neurologic symptoms, such as weakness, numbness and tingling, loss of bowel or bladder function, and sexual dysfunction, which may indicate cauda equina syndrome, which requires urgent surgical decompression.[30] Plain film radiographs of the lumbar spine in AP and lateral views can identify intervertebral narrowing, spondylolisthesis, osteophytes, vertebral height loss, and some fractures that indicate a lumbar spine origin of the hip pain. Lumbar MRI provides more specificity in identifying the root cause of the patient's pain. Referral to an orthopedic spine specialist or neurologist is recommended for further evaluation and management when conservative measures fail.

Hip Joint Infection

In contrast to the acute pain scenario, when hip pain has an insidious onset over a few days or weeks, questions should follow, such as, "Have you had any recent procedures or infections?" History of hip arthroplasty, immunocompromise, and/or diabetes is also important and can lead to the diagnosis of septic arthritis of the hip. Most often, these patients are older and admit to recent systemic symptoms of fever and chills, malaise, and sometimes are able to identify a nidus of infection, such as an open wound or ulcer. Rarely, recent extensive dental surgery or oral infection is the source of septic arthritis, especially in the setting of a hip arthroplasty.

Examination may reveal redness, swelling, or warmth around the hip joint; pain with range of motion of the hip in all planes; and significant antalgic gait. Initial work-up of the suspected acute septic hip joint includes a hip radiograph, which may be negative or may demonstrate a fluid collection; a hip aspiration for fluid to be sent for analysis; and bloodwork to identify an elevated white count with left shift, elevated C-reactive protein, elevated erythrocyte sedimentation rate, and positive culture for bacteria. MRI of the hip further demonstrates signs of infection including synovial enhancement, perisynovial edema, and joint effusion.[31] These findings are of critical importance to be identified quickly and the patient should be urgently referred for further treatment by an orthopedist (**Fig. 3**).

SUMMARY

Hip pain is a common complaint in adult patients. Because of the high frequency of complaints, it is essential for all clinicians to have a guide in assessing these patients. Asking the most pertinent questions in the appropriate order leads the clinician to the most common diagnoses that can, in many instances, be treated with conservative management, as outlined previously. Descriptive, open-ended inquiries paint a more accurate diagnostic picture than "yes-no" questions, and although all hip pain scenarios are not the same, the similarities narrow the diagnosis, which can then be further delineated with examination and testing. Listening carefully to patients' answers often guides the conversation and carves a clear path for the examination, testing, diagnosis, treatment, and possible referral to then follow. Consider this article a guide for the questions to be asked, which then lead to the most common causes of hip pain, rather than an all-inclusive path to all hip pain diagnoses. When these questions are coupled with careful listening skills, they can support the patient and the clinician in assessing, diagnosing, and treating the most common causes of hip pain while simultaneously bringing to light the more unusual sources of hip pain through the process of elimination.

CLINICS CARE POINTS

- Practitioners must listen to how hip pain is affecting patients in their daily life to direct questions toward a diagnosis.

- Open-ended questions elicit more diagnostic information.
- Hip pain described as "night-time pain" may lead to diagnoses including greater trochanteric pain syndrome (GTPS), osteoarthritis (OA), femoroacetabular impingement (FAI), avascular necrosis (AVN), and adult AVN or OA related to Legg-Calve-Perthes or slipped capital femoral epiphysis (SCFE).
- Hip pain described as "daytime pain with activity" may lead to diagnoses including soft tissue sprain or strain, acute or stress fracture of the hip, and labral tear.
- Hip pain described as "constant pain day and night" may lead to diagnoses including lumbar nerve impingement, sacroiliitis, and septic arthritis of the hip.

DISCLOSURES

None.

REFERENCES

1. Christmas C, Crespo CJ, Franckowiak SC, et al. How common is hip pain among older adults? Results from the Third National Health and Nutrition Examination Survey. J Fam Pract 2002;51(4):345–8.
2. Cecchi F, Mannoni A, Molino-Lova R, et al. Epidemiology of hip and knee pain in a community-based sample of Italian persons aged 65 and older. Osteoarthritis Cartilage 2008;16:1039.
3. Burnett RS, Della Rocca GJ, Prather H, et al. Clinical presentation of patients with tears of the acetabular labrum. J Bone Joint Surg Am 2006;88:1448.
4. Nunley RM, Prather H, Hunt D, et al. Clinical presentation of symptomatic acetabular dysplasia in skeletally mature patients. J Bone Joint Surg Am 2011;93(Suppl 2):17.
5. Thorborg K, Rathleff MS, Petersen P, et al. Prevalence and severity of hip and groin pain in sub-elite male football: a cross-sectional cohort study of 695 players. Scand J Med Sci Sports 2017;27:107.
6. Langhout R, Weir A, Litjes W, et al. Hip and groin injury is the most common non-time-loss injury in female amateur football. Knee Surg Sports Traumatol Arthrosc 2019;27:3133.
7. Chamberlain R. Hip pain in adults: evaluation and differential diagnosis. Am Fam Physician 2021;103(2):81–9.
8. Margo K. Evaluation and management of hip pain: an algorithmic approach. J Fam Pract 2003;52(8):607–17.
9. Poultsides LA, Bedi A, Kelly BT. An algorithmic approach to mechanical hip pain. HSS J 2012;8(3):213–24.
10. Tibor LM, Sekiya JK. Differential diagnosis of pain around the hip joint. Arthroscopy 2008;24(12):1407–21.
11. Segal NA, Felson DT, Torner JC, et al. Greater trochanteric pain syndrome: epidemiology and associated factors. Arch Phys Med Rehabil 2007;88:988.
12. Hunter D, Bierma-Zeinstra S. Osteoarthritis. Lancet 2019;393(10182):1745–59.
13. Murphy L, Helmick CG. The impact of osteoarthritis in the United States: a population-health perspective. Am J Nurs 2012;112(3 suppl 1):S13–9.
14. Fu M, Zhou H, Li Y, et al. Global, regional, and national burdens of hip osteoarthritis from 1990 to 2019: estimates from the 2019 Global Burden of Disease Study. Arthritis Res Ther 2022;24:8.
15. Gold G, Cicuttini F, Crema M, et al. OARSI Clinical Trials Recommendations: hip imaging in clinical trials in osteoarthritis. Osteoarthritis Cartilage 2015;23(5):716–31.

16. Dickenson E, Wall PD, Robinson B, et al. Prevalence of cam hip shape morphology: a systematic review. Osteoarthritis Cartilage 2016;24(6):949.
17. Cui L, Zhuang Q, Lin J, et al. Multicentric epidemiologic study on six thousand three hundred and ninety-five cases of femoral head osteonecrosis in China. Int Orthop 2016;40(2):267.
18. Shah KN, Racine J, Jones LC, et al. Pathophysiology and risk factors for osteonecrosis. Curr Rev Musculoskelet Med 2015;8(3):201–9.
19. Hauzeur JP, Pasteels JL, Schoutens A, et al. The diagnostic value of magnetic resonance imaging in non-traumatic osteonecrosis of the femoral head. J Bone Joint Surg Am 1989;71(5):641.
20. Mankin HJ. Nontraumatic necrosis of bone (osteonecrosis). N Engl J Med 1992; 326(22):1473–9.
21. Leunig M, Werlen S, Ungersbock A, et al. Evaluation of the acetabulum labrum by MR arthrography. J Bone Joint Surg Br 1997;79:230–4.
22. Narvani AA, Tsiridis E, Tai CC, et al. Acetabular labrum and its tears. Br J Sports Med 2003;37:207–11.
23. Schroeder J, Turner S, Buck E. Hip fractures: diagnosis and management. Am Fam Physician 2022;106(6):675–83.
24. Arlachov Y, Ibrahem Adam R. Acute hip pain: mimics of a femoral neck fracture. Clin Radiol 2018;73(9):773–81.
25. Wright AA, Hegedus EJ, Lenchik L, et al. Diagnostic accuracy of various imaging modalities for suspected lower extremity stress fractures: a systematic review with evidence-based recommendations for clinical practice. Am J Sports Med 2016;44(1):255–63.
26. Rubin DI. Epidemiology and risk factors for spine pain. Neurol Clin 2007;25(2): 353–71.
27. Buckland A, Miyamoto R, Patel R, et al. Differentiating hip pathology from lumbar spine pathology: key points of evaluation and management. J Am Acad Orthop Surg 2017;25:e23–34.
28. Hall S, Bartleson JD, Onofrio BM, et al. Lumbar spinal stenosis. Clinical features, diagnostic procedures, and results of surgical treatment in 68 patients. Ann Intern Med 1985;103:271.
29. Suri P, Rainville J, Katz J, et al. The accuracy of the physical examination for the diagnosis of midlumbar and low lumbar nerve root impingement. Spine 2011; 36(1):63–73.
30. Wagner R, Jagoda A. Spinal cord syndromes. Emerg Med Clin North Am 1997; 15:699.
31. Karchevsky M, Schweitzer M, Morrison W, et al. MRI findings of septic arthritis and associated osteomyelitis in adults. Am J of Roentgenology 2004;182:119–22.

Osteoarthritis of the Knee

Jodiann Williams, PA-C, MSPA[a], Kerby Pierre-Louis, MSPAS, PA-C[b],*

KEYWORDS

- Knee osteoarthritis • Knee pain • Knee osteoarthritis management
- Knee osteoarthritis risk factors

KEY POINTS

- Knee osteoarthritis affects 1 in 4 adults in the United States.
- X-rays are the preferred and initial imaging used to diagnose knee osteoarthritis.
- Risk factors for knee osteoarthritis include family history, overuse, obesity/overweight, and aging.
- Treatment for osteoarthritis is multifactorial and can include conservative or surgical treatment.
- In the surgical treatment of knee osteoarthritis, optimal outcomes are related to monitoring key factors such as body mass index, hemoglobin, nutritional status, and metabolic levels.

INTRODUCTION

Osteoarthritis and rheumatoid arthritis are the 2 most common types of arthritis and affect over 32.5 million American adults according to the Centers for Disease and Control and Prevention (CDC).[1] Osteoarthritis is inflammation of the joints. It is more commonly seen in adults and typically caused by degeneration of the cartilage. Subsequently, this leads to injury, deformity, and pain of the bones that make up that specific joint. The most common cause of this degeneration is the classic "wear and tear" of the joint from the many daily activities people carry out in their respective lives for work, school activities, recreational activities, and for sports and fitness activities. This type of arthritis can affect many joints but for this article, we will focus on osteoarthritis of the knee joint.[1]

According to the CDC between 2016 and 2018, around 1 in 4 adults in the United States were diagnosed with arthritis by a physician. This is the equivalent of around 58.5 million people. Arthritis was more commonly found in women at a rate of 24.7% in comparison to men, at a rate of 20.0%. Of the patients suffering from arthritis, 51.2% were described as having fair/poor health (pre-existing comorbidities such as heart disease, diabetes, and obesity) and 15.2% were in excellent/very good

a ARC Orthopedic Group, 7230 Medical Center Drive Suite 604, West Hills, CA 91307, USA;
b Acute Care Orthopedics
* Corresponding author. 7230 Medical Center Drive Suite 604, West Hills, CA 91307.
E-mail address: kerbypl@gmail.com

Physician Assist Clin 9 (2024) 59–69
https://doi.org/10.1016/j.cpha.2023.08.003
2405-7991/24/© 2023 Elsevier Inc. All rights reserved.

physicianassistant.theclinics.com

health (no pre-existing comorbidities and maintains active lifestyle). Studies show that the prevalence of arthritis was highest among adults with no physical activity (30.9%) when compared with adults who have limited activity (27%) or those who maintain/meet appropriate physical activity requirements (18.8%).[2]

Anatomy of the Knee

The knee is the largest joint of the body and is commonly affected by osteoarthritis.[3] The anatomy of the knee is made up of 3 bones: the femur, patella, and tibia. The femur is a long bone in which the proximal side helps form the hip joint and the distal end forms the superior aspect of the knee joint. The tibia, another long bone, comprises the lower part of the knee joint. The tibia's proximal side forms the inferior aspect of the knee joint and the distal side forms the superior part of the ankle, along with the distal end of the fibula. The patella is the final skeletal structure of the knee joint and this bone sits in front of the femur and tibia and allows for flexion and extension of the knee. Flexion and extension of the knee is necessary to walk, run, jump, kneel, and assists in many other functional movements we carry out on a daily basis.[4]

Outside of the bones that make up the knee joint, there is soft tissue called cartilage (specifically the distal femoral articular cartilage, patellar cartilage, medial meniscus, and lateral meniscus) that serves as a protective barrier for the femur, patella, and tibia. This protective barrier provides cushioning to support the movements of the knee so that there is no pain as they absorb majority of the impact and stress placed on the knees. The distal femoral articular cartilage wraps around the distal femoral cortex while the patellar cartilage is found on the posterior side of the patella and the menisci (medial and lateral), popularly known as the "shock absorbers" of the knee, sit on top of the tibia and take the majority of impact from the knee movements.

The remaining major anatomic structures of the knee include the synovial membrane and the knee ligaments. The synovial membrane is largely responsible for the frictionless movement of the knee. It lines the surfaces of the joint and produces synovial fluid. The synovial fluid allows the joint to move smoothly without friction. The major knee ligaments include the medial collateral ligament (MCL), the lateral collateral ligament (LCL), the posterior cruciate ligament (PCL), and the anterior cruciate ligament (ACL). These ligaments help to stabilize the knee. The MCL lines the medial compartment of the knee and helps resist valgus stress placed on the knee. The MCL originates from the proximal and posterior region of the medial femoral epicondyle. Out of all the ligaments of the knee, the MCL has the most complex anatomic makeup. The MCL is made of different layers identified as the superficial and deep layers. The superficial layer of the MCL is considered the most important structure for stabilization of the medial knee. The superficial MCL layer has 2 insertions on the tibia in which the proximal portion attaches distal to the plateau articular surface by about 12 mm, and the distal portion inserts distal to the joint line by about 6 mm. The deep layer of the MCL is identified as the thicker part of the MCL and originates from the middle third of the medial knee capsule. The deep layer of the MCL has 2 arms that are called the meniscofemoral and meniscotibial arms and they attach the medial meniscus to the joint capsule.[5] The LCL originates on the lateral epicondyle of the femur and it inserts on the fibular head.[6] The PCL sits in between the distal femur and proximal tibia and originates from the anterolateral aspect of the medial femoral condyle within the notch and inserts along the posterior aspect of the tibial plateau.[7] This ligament prevents the tibia from translating or shifting posteriorly. The ACL originates at the medial wall of the lateral femoral condyle and inserts into the middle of the intercondylar area.[8] The ACL sits next to the PCL and prevents the tibia from translating or shifting anteriorly.[9] A tear in the ACL is a commonly seen in athletes.

RISK FACTORS/DEMOGRAPHICS

Osteoarthritis can affect anyone and is irreversible once present. There are specific determinants and variables that can increase the chance of a patient developing knee osteoarthritis. **Table 1** lists these determinants and variables based on the age group of the patient.

Knee osteoarthritis can occur due to primary or secondary causes. A primary cause is a disorder that directly leads to osteoarthritis. A common primary cause of osteoarthritis is aging because as we get older, the joint naturally begins to experience degeneration causing osteoarthritis. A secondary cause is a consequence or an effect stemming from a primary cause of osteoarthritis. **Table 2** outlines common secondary causes of knee osteoarthritis.

HISTORY

Obtaining a detailed and thorough history is essential in diagnosing and therefore treating accurately. History should include onset of pain (insidious or sudden), duration of pain, specific location of knee pain (medial, lateral, anterior, posterior), character of pain (such as dull, aching, sharp), and whether there is any radiation of pain. Other important information to obtain includes the presence or absence of alleviating factors (such as icing, resting, medication, external support) and aggravating factors (such as walking, weight bearing, stair climbing). Specific information regarding whether activities of daily living, such as getting dressed or getting in and out of a car, are painful or limited should also be obtained. Assessing whether such activities and or exercising requires altering or modifications due to knee pain should also be noted. It is important to also obtain information on any attempted treatments and their timing thus far as this will aid in preparing an appropriate and effective treatment plan. Inquiring about any additional joint pains is imperative as this could indicate other inflammatory conditions. Careful attention should be paid to the history as knee pain can be referred from the lumbar spine or the hip joint.[10] The presence or absence of mechanical symptoms such as locking or catching during specific knee movement should be noted. Knee effusion may be present with knee osteoarthritis; therefore, the onset of effusion should be established.[11] The presence of effusion may indicate osteoarthritis or other acute injuries.

Osteoarthritis is a progressive disease, and not only involves the joint lining but also the cartilage, ligaments, and bone.[12] Patients with osteoarthritis primarily complain of knee pain with varying severity. Pain is most commonly related to activity level and is

Table 1 Common risk factors for osteoarthritis	
Adults	**Young Adults**
Menopause $\geq$ 50 y	Previous injury of the joint
Age	Congenital deformity
Overweight/obesity	Abnormal development of joint
Prior injury (to include surgery)	Genetic defect of joint cartilage
Repetitive overuse or cumulative injury (wear and tear)	
Family history of osteoarthritis	

Adapted from: Niams health information on osteoarthritis. National Institute of Arthritis and Musculoskeletal and Skin Diseases. https://www.niams.nih.gov/health-topics/osteoarthritis. Published June 8, 2022. Accessed April 15, 2023.

Table 2 Common secondary causes of knee osteoarthritis		
Surgical/Trauma	**Anatomic**	**Metabolic**
Posttraumatic	Congenital or malformation of the limb	Rickets
Postsurgical	Malposition (varus/valgus)	Rheumatoid arthritis
Avascular necrosis	Scoliosis	Acromegaly
Infectious arthritis	Paget disease	Menopause $\geq$ 50 y
Psoriatic arthritis	Chondrocalcinosis	Hemochromatosis
Sickle cell disease	Ochronosis	Gout/pseudogout Hemophilia Wilson's disease

Adapted from: Hsu H, Siwiec RM. Knee osteoarthritis. National Center for Biotechnology Information. https://pubmed.ncbi.nlm.nih.gov/29939661/. Published January 2023. Accessed April 15, 2023.

usually relieved by rest. Depending on severity of disease, knee pain may persist at rest as well. Cardinal symptoms of knee osteoarthritis include knee pain, reduced function, stiffness, joint instability, decreased range of motion, and deformity.[13] Location of knee pain may vary and usually correlates to findings on imaging study. Knee pain may be located medially, laterally, or anteriorly. It is often described as dull and constant in character that is exacerbated with activity and is often of gradual onset with associated knee swelling.[10] Reduced function secondary to knee pain generally increases as disease progresses affecting activities of daily living. Knee joint stiffness also progresses which results in decreased range of motion.

Physical Examination

The physical examination initially starts with complete visualization of the knee. If possible, the patient's gait should be examined as they ambulate in and around the examination room. Observation should focus on signs of pain or abnormal movement which can indicate ligamentous instability.[10] Inspection includes identifying edema, deformity, erythema, and the condition of surrounding skin, such as whether it is intact or has a dermatologic condition or the presence of any scars. One specific deformity that is important to observe for is misalignment of the knees. If present, differentiate between Genu varus and Genu valgum. Assessment of range of motion is an essential component of the physical examination as deficits can limit patient function and or mobility. Range of motion is measured in degrees and used to assess extension and flexion of the knee. The normal range is 0° of extension to 140° of flexion. Palpation of the knee and surrounding structures is performed to assess for areas of tenderness and for the presence of nonvisible deformities. The special knee tests used to further assess the structures of the knee include Ely's test, Ober test, Lachman's, posterior Sag, Varus at 30°, Valgus at 0/30, McMurray's, Apley's, Waldron sign, grind test, and vastus medialis oblique test.[14]

Imaging Studies

X-rays are the most common imaging modality used to diagnose knee osteoarthritis. It also serves as a vital tool for monitoring its progression. The anterior-posterior view (AP) is typically the most helpful view for diagnostic purposes. Although X-rays are great for providing detail of the skeletal structures, they are not optimal for providing detailed information into possible surrounding or contributing soft tissue injury.[3] Radiographic findings can be correlated to anatomic changes (**Table 3**), but these

Table 3	
Common radiographic finding in knee osteoarthritis	
Anatomic Changes	**Radiographic Changes**
Medial tibiofemoral joint narrowing	Subchondral new bone formation
Patellofemoral joint narrowing	Osteophyte formation: Medial joint space
Lateral subluxation of the tibia can occur	Osteophyte formation: Anteromedial distal femur
Cartilage degeneration	Osteophyte formation: Anteromedial proximal tibia
Cartilage loss	Osteophyte formation: Lateral joint space
Subchondral bone formation	

Adapted from: Daniel L. Swagerty J, Hellinger D. Radiographic assessment of osteoarthritis. American Family Physician. https://www.aafp.org/pubs/afp/issues/2001/0715/p279.html. Published July 15, 2001. Accessed April 15, 2023.

findings are not always found.[9] However, when found, the severity of the osteoarthritis can be described and placed in different severity categories. The Kellgren-Lawrence (KL) classification system is often used and is the most broadly accepted method of classifying radiographic osteoarthritis. The system was originally described using AP radiographs, with grades assigned from 0 to 4.[15] The classification of the KL system is outlined below.[16]

Grade 1: Doubtful narrowing of knee joint space with possible osteophyte formation.
Grade 2: Possible narrowing of joint space with definite osteophyte formation.
Grade 3: Definite narrowing of joint space, moderate osteophyte formation, some sclerosis, possible bone deformity.
Grade 4: Severe narrowing of joint space, large osteophyte formation, marked sclerosis, definite deformity of bone ends.

Table 3 outlines anatomic changes in correlation with radiographic changes. These findings collectively or individually are not found in every X-ray.

MRI can also be used in diagnosing and evaluating knee osteoarthritis as it can provide more extensive detail into potential soft tissue contributing factors. With this tool, contributing diagnoses such as chondromalacia, meniscal tearing (acute vs traumatic vs degenerative), stress fracture, neoplasms, avascular necrosis, and others can be identified and thus provide a more complete understanding of a patient's specific diagnosis.[3]

Conservative Treatment

Treatment for knee osteoarthritis is multifactorial and can include conservative measures as well as surgical intervention.[17] Conservative measures are often attempted first. **Table 4** gives an overview of some conservative, nonarthroplasty treatment options and their recommendation grade. Conservative measures include the use of external support, such as a knee brace, walker, canes, or shoe insole, along with other nonpharmacologic treatments such as exercise, diet, and weight loss if applicable, physical therapy, and other alternative treatments. These options may aid in the relief of knee pain due to osteoarthritis. There are several pharmacologic agents available in the treatment of osteoarthritis including anti-inflammatory medications. Anti-inflammatory medications may be over the counter in the form of topical creams/gel/patch or in the form of oral capsules/tablets. An option for topical treatment

Table 4
Management of knee pain due to osteoarthritis (nonarthroplasty)[15,18–20]

Types of Conservative Interventions	Treatment/Management	Recommendation Grade
Self-Management/ Patient Education	Advising patient on accurate management and understanding of knee osteoarthritis including thorough treatment options and medication adherence	Strong
Dietary/joint supplements	Turmeric	Limited
	Ginger Extract	Limited
	Glucosamine	Limited
	Chondroitin	Limited
	Vitamin D	Limited
	Weight Loss	Moderate
Conservative external support	Cane	Moderate
	Knee brace	Moderate
	Lateral wedge insole	Not recommended
Exercise	Supervised	Strong
	Aquatic	Strong
Manual/Physical therapy	Massage	Limited
	TENS	Limited
	Percutaneous Electrical Nerve Stimulation	Limited
	Neuromuscular Training	Moderate
	Extracorporeal shockwave therapy	Limited
	Manual therapy	Low
	Mobilization, manual traction, passive range of motion	Not studied
	Myofascial release treatment	NG
Alternative treatment	Acupuncture	Low
	Tai Chi Mind Body Therapy	NG
	Thermal modalities (heat/cold)	
	Laser therapy- Low level laser therapy (LLLT)	
	Therapeutic ultrasound	
	Kinesio taping	
	Cannabidiol treatment	
Medications	Oral NSAIDS	Strong
	Topical NSAIDS	Strong
	Oral Acetaminophen	Strong
	Oral Narcotics	Not recommended
	Oral SSRIs and SNRIs for chronic pain	Not studied
	Gabapentin	Not studied
Conservative - Needles	Hyaluronic Acid	Not recommended
	Acupuncture	Limited
	Intraarticular Corticosteroids	Moderate
	Platelet rich plasma	Limited
	Dry Needling	No supporting evidence

(continued on next page)

Table 4 (continued)		
Types of Conservative Interventions	Treatment/Management	Recommendation Grade
Surgical	Laser treatment	Limited
	Denervation therapy	Limited
	Lavage/debridement	Not recommended
	Partial meniscectomy*	Moderate
	Tibial osteotomy	Limited
	Free floating interpositional devices	No supporting evidence

Abbreviations: AAOS, American Academy of Orthopedic Surgeons; TENS, Transcutaneous Electrical Nerve Stimulation; NSAIDS, Nonsteroidal anti-inflammatory drugs; RX-treatment, PT-physical therapy; NG-not graded, * done for secondary treatment to remove torn meniscus with mild to moderate osteoarthritis in those who have failed physical therapy or other nonsurgical treatments.

Adapted from: American Academy of Orthopaedic Surgeons Management of Osteoarthritis of the Knee (Non-Arthroplasty) Evidence-Based Clinical Practice Guideline (3rd Edition). https://www.aaos.org/oak3cpg Published August 31, 2021. Accessed April 15, 2023.

includes diclofenac, a nonsteroidal anti-inflammatory drug (NSAIDs).[21] Other pharmacologic agents that can be used for myofacial pain include topical creams such as Bengay ultra strength muscle pain ointment, Biofreeze, and Icy Hot extra strength cream.[22] If these initial measures provide an inadequate response, there are several types of intra-articular treatments available including intra-articular steroid injections, intra-articular hyaluronic acid injections, and platelet rich plasma injections.

Knee osteoarthritis may lead to chronic pain. Chronic pain is defined as ongoing pain lasting longer than 6 months, and it continues to be a leading health care cost burden in the United States.[23] Pain medications are the mainstay to treat chronic pain; however, other classes of drugs can be used in certain circumstances. Anti-depressants may assist in pain management where pain sensitization is present.[24] Serotonin noradrenaline reuptake inhibitors (SNRIs) have been used to treat a range of musculoskeletal pain conditions, expanding from everyday use for depressive disorders.[23] SNRIs including duloxetine, venlafaxine, and milnacipran have demonstrated efficacy in reducing pain in musculoskeletal pain-osteoarthritis.[23] Gabapentin has been shown to be effective in reducing pain in knee osteoarthritis.[25] Cannabidiol is a nonpsychoactive cannabinoid that has shown promise in preclinical studies to reduce inflammation and pain associated with arthritis.[26] Delta-9-tetrahydrocannabinol has well-established effects on pain but is associated with psychoactive effects that may hinder its application in the pain reduction setting.[26]

Surgical Treatment

Total knee arthroplasty (TKA), also referred to as total knee replacement, is a surgical treatment option for patients with knee osteoarthritis who have failed conservative treatment measures. It is an effective procedure that provides pain relief and improves the patient's functional status.[27] The demand for TKA in the United States is anticipated to increase 673% from 2005 to 2030, with 5.28 million TKAs being done annually.[28]

Being an elective procedure, the determination of proceeding with a TKA is primarily based on symptoms combined with radiologic findings. The minimum requirements for total TKA are significant, prolonged symptoms with supporting clinical and radiological signs.[27] The contraindications for TKA are an active infection or a medically unstable patient. There are several factors that should be considered to minimize complications for patients undergoing a TKA. The patient's hemoglobin level is an important factor pre- and postoperatively. Blood management strategy, that is monitoring and planning for blood loss prior to surgery, can be directly related to patient outcome. Options for maximizing hemoglobin level in preparation for TKA include iron supplements, which can be given orally or intravenously, and erythropoietin.[29] Another factor to consider is the use of tranexamic acid (TXA), a fibrinolysis inhibitor, which prevents clot lysis by blocking the proteolytic activity of plasminogen activators.[30] TXA can be used, although not standard of care, and has shown in preliminary studies to aid in the reduction of blood loss with a TKA.[30] The patient's nutritional status is another factor that bears consideration. Measurement of serum albumin, prealbumin, transferrin, and total lymphocyte count can be used to identify at-risk patients for preoperative malnutrition.[31] TKA patients clinically found to be malnourished have demonstrated worse postoperative outcomes including prolonged hospital stay, require additional surgeries, increased rates of infection, and increased mortality rates.[31] Nasal *Staphylococcus aureus* screening and decolonization has been widely used to reduce surgical site infections prior to total knee and hip arthroplasty.[32] History of smoking was associated with an increased risk of medical complications, increased analgesia usage, and higher mortality following arthroplasty.[33] Therefore, smoking cessation discussion and counseling is imperative in surgical planning. These factors when considered and managed appropriately can assist in minimizing complications for patients undergoing TKA.

Besides a TKA, additional surgical treatment options are currently available for the treatment of knee osteoarthritis. These other surgical treatments include, but not limited to, arthroscopic lavage and debridement and unicompartmental knee arthroplasty (UKA). Arthroscopic lavage and debridement is a procedure done to attempt repair of the rough cartilage and degenerative meniscus; however, studies fail to demonstrate significant benefit in treating knee osteoarthritis.[34] Unicompartmental knee arthroplasty is used when osteoarthritis is limited to one compartment of the knee and involves replacing the contact surfaces of the affected compartment with a prothesis. Although a UKA is less invasive, it has a limited indication and has an inferior long-term survival rate (80.2%–98% at 10 years) in comparison to TKA (98% at 15 years).[34]

SUMMARY

Osteoarthritis of the knee is one of the most common forms of arthritis and is increasing in prevalence. It can be extremely painful and disabling for patients. The importance of understanding knee anatomy significantly aids with examination and accurate diagnosis. Being familiar with common risk factors helps with accurate diagnosing and patient counseling/education. A thorough history and physical examination is vital to the accurate assessment of patients. X-rays are the preferred and most commonly used diagnostic imaging tool for knee osteoarthritis. The treatments for knee osteoarthritis continue to evolve and include several types of conservative measures and surgical interventions for improved quality of life for affected patients.

CLINICS CARE POINTS

- Obese patients, individuals with chronic high stress/overuse activity, and individuals with very sedentary lifestyles are at higher risk for osteoarthritis.

- Knee osteoarthritis, once present, is irreversible but with appropriate conservative therapy and reduced heavy stress to the joint, the progression may be delayed substantially.
- Some common conservative measures of knee osteoarthritis treatment include low impact exercise (stationary bicycle, elliptical, swimming/aqua therapy etc.), NSAIDs, cortisone and/or hyaluronic gel intra-articular injections, physical therapy, and knee support bracing.
- End-stage management of knee osteoarthritis is a total knee replacement for patients who fit the criteria for surgical intervention based on the surgeon's professional assessment.

DISCLOSURE

The authors have nothing to disclose.

REFERENCES

1. Osteoarthritis (OA). Centers for Disease Control and Prevention. https://www.cdc.gov/arthritis/basics/osteoarthritis.htm. Published July 27, 2020. Accessed April 15, 2023.
2. National statistics. Centers for Disease Control and Prevention. https://www.cdc.gov/arthritis/data_statistics/national-statistics.html. Published October 12, 2021. Accessed July 19, 2023.
3. Frassica FJ, Sponseller PD, Wilckens JH, et al. Knee Pain; Osteoarthritis. In: The 5-minute orthopaedic consult. 2nd ed. Philadelphia, PA: Wolters Kluwer; 2007. p. 218–85.
4. Sheth NP, Foran JRH. Arthritis of the knee - orthoinfo - aaos. OrthoInfo. https://orthoinfo.aaos.org/en/diseases–conditions/arthritis-of-the-knee/. Published July 14, 2020. Accessed April 15, 2023. Peer Reviewed by Stuart J. Fischer, MD, FAAOS. Last Reviewed: February 2023.
5. Vosoughi F, Rezaei Dogahe R, Nuri A, Ayati Firoozabadi M, Mortazavi J. Medial collateral ligament injury of the knee: A review on current concept and Management. The archives of bone and joint surgery. https://www.ncbi.nlm.nih.gov/pmc/articles/PMC8221433/. Published May 2021. Accessed April 16, 2023.
6. Yaras RJ, O'Neill N, Yaish AM. Lateral collateral ligament knee injuries - statpearls - NCBI bookshelf. NIH National Library of Medicine. https://www.ncbi.nlm.nih.gov/books/NBK560847/. Published January 2023. Accessed April 16, 2023.
7. Logterman SL, Wydra FB, Frank RM. Posterior cruciate ligament: Anatomy and biomechanics. Current Reviews in Musculoskeletal Medicine 2018;11(3):510–4.
8. Petersen W, Tillmann B. Anatomie und Funktion des Vorderen Kreuzbandes. Orthopä 2002;31(8):710–8.
9. Daniel L. Swagerty J, Hellinger D. Radiographic assessment of osteoarthritis. American Family Physician. https://www.aafp.org/pubs/afp/issues/2001/0715/p279.html. Published July 15, 2001. Accessed April 15, 2023.
10. Hsu H, Siwiec RM. Knee osteoarthritis. National Center for Biotechnology Information. https://pubmed.ncbi.nlm.nih.gov/29939661/. Published January 2023. Accessed April 15, 2023.
11. Calmbach WL, Hutchens M. Evaluation of patients presenting with knee pain: Part I. History, physical examination, radiographs, and laboratory tests. Am Fam Physician 2003;68(5):907–12.
12. Alshami AM. Knee osteoarthritis related pain: a narrative review of diagnosis and treatment. Int J Health Sci 2014;8(1):85–104.

13. Hunter DJ, McDougall JJ, Keefe FJ. The symptoms of osteoarthritis and the genesis of pain. Rheum Dis Clin North Am 2008;34(3):623–43.

14. Iversen MD, Price LL, von Heideken J, et al. Physical examination findings and their relationship with performance-based function in adults with knee osteoarthritis. BMC Musculoskelet Disord 2016;17:273.

15. Kohn MD, Sassoon AA, Fernando ND. Classifications in Brief: Kellgren-Lawrence Classification of Osteoarthritis. Clin Orthop Relat Res 2016;474(8):1886–93.

16. KELLGREN JH, LAWRENCE JS. Radiological assessment of osteo-arthrosis. Ann Rheum Dis 1957;16(4):494–502.

17. American Academy of Orthopaedic Surgeons Management of Osteoarthritis of the Knee (NonArthroplasty) Evidence-Based Clinical Practice Guideline. https://www.aaos.org/oak3cpg Published August 30, 2021.

18. Wang C. Complementary and Alternative Medicine and Osteoarthritis. Int J Integr Med 2013;1:13.

19. Dantas LO, Salvini TF, McAlindon TE. Knee osteoarthritis: key treatments and implications for physical therapy. Braz J Phys Ther 2021;25(2):135–46.

20. Dor A, Kalichman L. A myofascial component of pain in knee osteoarthritis. J Bodyw Mov Ther 2017;21(3):642–7.

21. Bariguian Revel F, Fayet M, Hagen M. Topical Diclofenac, an Efficacious Treatment for Osteoarthritis: A Narrative Review. Rheumatol Ther 2020;7(2):217–36.

22. Avrahami D, Hammond A, Higgins C, et al. A randomized, placebo-controlled double-blinded comparative clinical study of five over-the-counter non-pharmacological topical analgesics for myofascial pain: single session findings. Chiropr Man Therap 2012;20:7.

23. Robinson C, Dalal S, Chitneni A, et al. A Look at Commonly Utilized Serotonin Noradrenaline Reuptake Inhibitors (SNRIs) in Chronic Pain. Health Psychol Res 2022;10(3):32309.

24. Leaney AA, Lyttle JR, Segan J, et al. Antidepressants for hip and knee osteoarthritis. Cochrane Database Syst Rev 2022;10(10):CD012157.

25. Enteshari-Moghaddam A, Azami A, Isazadehfar K, et al. Efficacy of duloxetine and gabapentin in pain reduction in patients with knee osteoarthritis. Clin Rheumatol 2019;38(10):2873–80.

26. Frane N, Stapleton E, Iturriaga C, et al. Cannabidiol as a treatment for arthritis and joint pain: an exploratory cross-sectional study. J Cannabis Res 2022;4(1):47.

27. Adie S, Harris I, Chuan A, et al. Selecting and optimising patients for total knee arthroplasty. Med J Aust 2019;210(3):135–41.

28. Shah A, Cieremans D, Slover J, et al. Trends in Complications and Outcomes in Patients Aged 65 Years and Younger Undergoing Total Knee Arthroplasty: Data From the American Joint Replacement Registry. J Am Acad Orthop Surg Glob Res Rev 2022;6(6):e2200116.

29. Liu D, Dan M, Martinez Martos S, et al. Blood Management Strategies in Total Knee Arthroplasty. Knee Surg Relat Res 2016;28(3):179–87.

30. Marra F, Rosso F, Bruzzone M, et al. Use of tranexamic acid in total knee arthroplasty. Joints 2017;4(4):202–13.

31. Dubé MD, Rothfusz CA, Emara AK, et al. Nutritional Assessment and Interventions in Elective Hip and Knee Arthroplasty: A Detailed Review and Guide to Management. Curr Rev Musculoskelet Med 2022;15(4):311–22.

32. Zhu X, Sun X, Zeng Y, et al. Can nasal Staphylococcus aureus screening and decolonization prior to elective total joint arthroplasty reduce surgical site and

prosthesis-related infections? A systematic review and meta-analysis. J Orthop Surg Res 2020;15(1):60.

33. Matharu GS, Mouchti S, Twigg S, et al. The effect of smoking on outcomes following primary total hip and knee arthroplasty: a population-based cohort study of 117,024 patients. Acta Orthop 2019;90(6):559–67.

34. Rönn K, Reischl N, Gautier E, et al. Current surgical treatment of knee osteoarthritis. Arthritis 2011;2011:454873.

Foot and Ankle Injuries with the Rise of Pickleball

Check for updates

Elise Elegeert, DMSC, MS, MAT, PA-C[a],*, Allison J. Justice, MMS, PA-C[a],
Robert Martin Shipman Sr, MHA, PA, CMCO[a], Aaron J. Guyer, MD[b],
Jason Beaver, MHS, MEd, PA-C[a]

KEYWORDS

- Pickleball injuries • Racket sports injuries • Plantar fasciitis • Achilles tendon rupture
- Achilles tendonitis • Fifth metatarsal fracture • Ankle fracture • Ankle sprains

KEY POINTS

- Below-knee injuries are the most common musculoskeletal injury seen in sports participation.
- Racket sport injuries illustrate some of the most common below-knee pathology.
- Pickleball is one of the fastest growing sports in the world, particularly among older individuals, and is becoming a frequent cause of common foot and ankle injuries.

INTRODUCTION

With a popularity growth rate of 158.6% over the previous 3 years,[1] pickleball should be something on the radar of all clinicians that work in a primary care, urgent care, or emergency setting, in addition to those in orthopedics and sports medicine (**Fig. 1**). Pickleball is a paddle sport that can be played either indoors or outdoors. It uses a smaller court than other racket sports, being only 20 feet by 44 feet and uses a lower net. It can be played individually or in doubles and uses a paddle that is between a ping-pong paddle and tennis racket in size and a ball with holes similar in size to a Wiffle ball.[2] Tennis, pickleball, and other racket sports have many similarities and differences in the rules, equipment, and court layout. These sports require quick movements and changes in direction which can put great stress on the lower extremities. Many injuries in these sports can be debilitating to the patient's quality of life and can even lead to time away from the sport itself or loss of work time.[3] The lower extremity injuries obtained in these sports, with a focus on pickleball, will be reviewed and discussed.

[a] Florida State University College of Medicine, School of Physician Assistant Practice, 1115 West Call Street, Suite G108, Tallahassee, FL 32306, USA; [b] Florida State University College of Medicine, Tallahassee Orthopedic Clinic, 3334 Capital Medical Boulevard, Suite 400, Tallahassee, FL 32317-3100, USA
* Corresponding author.
E-mail address: elise.elegeert@med.fsu.edu

Physician Assist Clin 9 (2024) 71–79
https://doi.org/10.1016/j.cpha.2023.07.008
2405-7991/24/© 2023 Elsevier Inc. All rights reserved.
physicianassistant.theclinics.com

Key Pickleball Stats for 2023

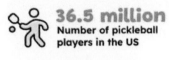

36.5 million
Number of pickleball
players in the US

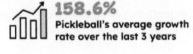

158.6%
Pickleball's average growth
rate over the last 3 years

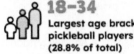

18–34
Largest age bracket of
pickleball players
(28.8% of total)

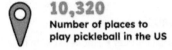

10,320
Number of places to
play pickleball in the US

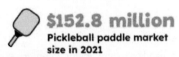

$152.8 million
Pickleball paddle market
size in 2021

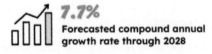

7.7%
Forecasted compound annual
growth rate through 2028

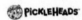

Fig. 1. Pickleball statistics. (Mackie B. Pickleball statistics: America's fastest growing sport in 2023. Pickleheads. https://www.pickleheads.com/blog/pickleball-statistics. Published February 24, 2023. Accessed April 30, 2023.)

These racket sports have many of the same types of injuries in common but may be different in the severity and complexity of the associated injury. One study found that pickleball-related injuries have been increasing in recent years compared with rates observed in other racket sports. The investigators also found that injuries seem to be tied to an older population but closely divided equally by sex.[2] The Sports and Fitness Industry Association estimated that there were 2.8 million people playing pickleball in 2017; the participants tended to be older, with 42% of all players over the age of 65 years.[2] **Box 1** lists the most common acute and chronic injuries seen below-the-knee that is associated with pickleball.[2] The evaluation, diagnosis, and treatment of each of these will be reviewed.

ACUTE INJURIES
Ankle Sprains and Fractures

Ankle injuries are common among athletes participating in a variety of sports and are especially common in indoor and court sports.[4] Lower extremity sprains and strains accounted for approximately 30% each of pickleball-related injuries in emergency departments in the United States from 2001 to 2017.[5] In pickleball, there is quick movement and turning on a point that can lead to inversion of the ankle causing sprains, especially in amateur athletes.[3]

Ankle "sprain" is a very broad term describing a continuum of injury, from stretching or partially tearing the ligamentous structures of the ankle, to complete tears and dislocations. It is the most common musculoskeletal injury seen in the primary care, emergency or urgent care setting, accounting for 75% of all ankle trauma, and 10% to 30% of sports injuries overall. There are over 1 million visits to primary care offices each year for ankle sprains.[6]

Box 1
Most common acute and chronic below-the-knee injuries associated with pickleball[2]

Acute Injuries
• Ankle sprain
• Ankle fracture
• Achilles tendon rupture
• Fifth metatarsal fracture

Chronic Injuries
• Achilles tendonitis
• Plantar fasciitis

Evaluation of a patient with an ankle injury should begin with a complete history and physical examination. The patient usually can describe the typical mechanism of ankle sprain, which is a plantar flexion or inversion injury. They will describe lateral pain and may, or may not, be able to bear weight. Occasionally, they will have a history of previous sprains or similar injury. Bruising and swelling is commonly present, and it is important to determine where the patient is tender.[6] Neurovascular evaluation is essential, including palpation of dorsalis pedis and posterior tibialis pulses, motor functions, and sensation of the injured limb, to rule out other more significant injuries. Understandably, patients may not give their full effort with motor function due to pain, but this attempt is to help determine the extent of the injury, whether it is disruption of bony structure or soft tissue injury.[6]

It is important to rule out fractures in ankle injuries as management may change drastically. Several guidelines have been developed to determine when radiographic evaluation is warranted. The Ottawa Ankle Rules are the most commonly used example (**Fig. 2**). Appropriate ankle x-rays include anterior–posterior (AP), lateral and mortise views, and appropriate foot x-rays include AP, lateral, and oblique views. Advanced imaging studies, such as MRI, are rarely indicated and should only be ordered by an orthopedic specialist.[6]

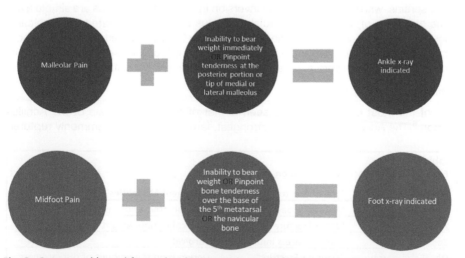

Fig. 2. Ottawa ankle and foot rules. (*Adapted from* Wolfe MW, et al. Management of ankle sprains. American Family Physician. 2001,63(1):93-104.)

The initial management of ankle sprains includes non- to light-weight-bearing, elective immobilization, rest, ice, compression, and elevation to reduce swelling.[3] Early protected weight-bearing and appropriate physical therapy techniques have been shown to accelerate healing time and can help to avoid chronic ankle instability. Cast boots and ankle braces are often needed, but casting should be avoided. Simple sprains and strains may take several weeks to improve and resolve, whereas more severe injuries can take 3 months or more.[3]

Chronic ankle instability can result after repetitive inversion type ankle sprains, especially if not treated appropriately. It is characterized by the ankle "giving way" throughout the day, or with athletic activity. Ligamentous laxity and proprioceptive deficits or muscle weakness lead to this problem, which emphasizes why early protected weight-bearing and physical therapy techniques are essential in preventing greater morbidity after an acute injury. In addition to neuromuscular and sensorimotor training, applying Kinesio tape may help reduce instability and improve ankle function after repetitive injuries.[4,7]

Patients should be referred to an orthopedic or sports medicine physician in specific situations. When a fracture or tendon rupture is suspected or diagnosed, immediate referral should be made. Patients with a suspected ankle sprain who fail the usual management outlined above, or have a history of recurrent sprains and ankle instability, warrant a consultation with a specialist as well.

Fractures of the Ankle and Foot

Proximal fifth metatarsal fracture is one of the most common foot injuries. It is often seen in jumping sports, as can be seen in tennis, pickleball, and basketball, in which the ankle is plantar flexed and inverted, resulting in a great force applied to the lateral metatarsals. The Jones fracture is a well-known eponym describing a fracture of the fifth metatarsal, but not all fifth metatarsal fractures are Jones fractures. The classification of these injuries is based on location of the fracture due to the varied blood supply to the fifth metatarsal.[8]

Location of the fracture is important as this determines treatment (**Table 1**). Referral to an orthopedic surgeon is essential if a zone 2, zone 3, or dancer's fracture is diagnosed.[9]

Ankle fractures can occur with sports such as pickleball with a mechanism similar to ankle sprains, with varying degrees of inversion injury. Some fractures are simple avulsions at the tip of the fibula or medial malleolus and can be treated nonsurgically. These simple avulsion fractures can be treated with Controlled Ankle Movement boots for 4 to 6 weeks with appropriate follow-up with an orthopedic specialist; other fractures that are more severe may require surgical interventions with a specialist.

Achilles Tendon Rupture

One of the most common injuries seen is that of a sprain or strain of the Achilles tendon.[5] The Achilles tendon is the strongest, largest, and most commonly ruptured

Table 1		
Fifth metatarsal fractures by location		
Fracture Location	**Type of Fracture**	**Treatment Modalities**
Zone 1	Metatarsal base fracture	Nonoperative with cast shoe/boot
Zone 2	"Jones Fracture"	Surgical or non-weight-bearing in a cast
Zone 3	Acute or stress injuries	Surgical
Distal metatarsal	"Dancer's Fracture"	Depends on the amount of displacement, occasionally surgical

tendon in the human body. In many cases, the rupture is acute and secondary to abrupt forces put on the tendon while active in a sport that requires running or with acute explosive push-offs,[10] such as what is done in pickleball. Occasionally, it can result from a chronic festering of ongoing debilitating Achilles tendinitis (discussed later).

Patients often give a history of an abrupt motion, usually pushing off, and then feeling a "pop" or hearing a loud noise. Afterward, they may have difficulty pushing off with that limb. Amazingly, pain is not always present.[10] Physical examination will demonstrate bruising and swelling around the posterior ankle and often a palpable defect can be found over the Achilles tendon. Comparing the injured and uninjured leg is essential, with the patient lying prone on the examination table. Pathognomonic findings include increased resting dorsi flexion of the injured foot, and a positive Thompson's test. This test is "positive" when squeezing of the affected limb fails to produce plantar flexion of the foot, whereas the patient is lying prone[10] (**Fig. 3**).

Imaging studies are not usually recommended because physical examination alone can define diagnosis. In rare cases, there may be some unequivocal findings in the physical examination, thus warranting MRI or ultrasound evaluation.[10] If an Achilles tendon rupture is suspected, the patient should be immobilized in plantar flexion and an immediate referral for consultation to an orthopedic specialist is warranted. Ongoing management post-immobilization may include physical therapy or possible surgical repair.[10]

CHRONIC AND OVERUSE CONDITIONS
Plantar Fasciitis

The plantar fascia is a thick fibrous band extending from the calcaneus to the metatarsal heads (**Fig. 4**). Among its many functions is the role it plays in pressure distribution and maintenance of the plantar arches. Plantar fasciitis a common injury which can occur from pickleball due to the repetitive, and sometimes excessive forces exerted on the feet during these matches, which involve sustained high-impact activity. Stretching of the plantar fascia due to this pressure can become symptomatic not only for newer participants to increased activity but also the well-conditioned athlete. Although the pathophysiology is not completely understood, recent evidence

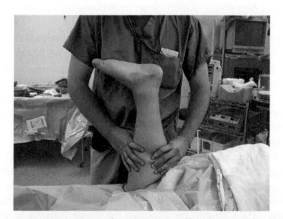

Fig. 3. Thompson's test. Squeezing of uninjured calf will produce foot plantarflexion, whereas calf squeeze of leg with ruptured Achilles will not (positive Thompson test). (Metzl JA, Ahmad CS, Levine WN. The ruptured Achilles tendon: operative and non-operative treatment options. *Curr Rev Musculoskelet Med.* 2008;1(2):161-164. https://doi.org/10.1007/s12178-008-9025-4.)

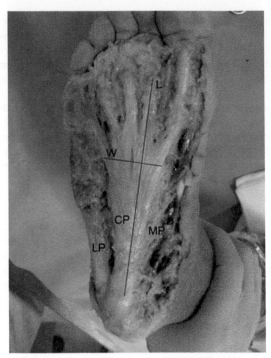

Fig. 4. Plantar fascia. (Chen D-w, Li B, Aubeeluck A, Yang Y-f, Huang Y-g, Zhou J-q, et al. (2014) Anatomy and Biomechanical Properties of the Plantar Aponeurosis: A Cadaveric Study. PLoS ONE 9(1): e84347. https://doi.org/10.1371/journal.pone.0084347.)

suggests that plantar fasciitis is due to a disruption in normal biomechanics that results in repetitive small tears in the plantar fascia.[11] As a result, the stiffening of the plantar fascia and subsequent inflammation can become symptomatic with the expression of heel pain that is greater after the completion of activity or extended periods of rest. For example, the patient may report that getting out of bed in the morning includes very painful first steps, which often improve with movement (as the plantar fascia begins to loosen).

The diagnosis of this condition is often clinically based revealing primarily plantar medial heel pain, which can include increased pain with dorsiflexion of the symptomatic foot. Imaging such as x-ray is not often necessary but could be considered to rule out any bony abnormalities which may be contributing to the symptoms. Physical examination may reveal a high plantar arch or flat foot associated with the condition. It is necessary to ensure that this is not related to other causes such as Achilles tendonitis, nerve entrapment, or calf tightness.

Treatment is strongly focused on nonoperative management, which revolves around rest, modification to lower impact activity, and stretches that target the plantar fascia and calf. Supportive shoes and heel inserts can make a remarkable difference. Splints that are worn at night are an option for many to maintain the stretch of these targeted areas overnight. Reducing the inflammation by using nonsteroidal anti-inflammatory drugs (NSAIDs) can be effective for those without contraindications to this medication. The application of ice to the foot is also an additional way to reduce inflammation, such as freezing a water-filled bottle then rolling it with the effected foot. Patient education that this condition may take 2 to 3 months to resolve with appropriate nonoperative treatments is imperative.

The failure of these initial treatments should prompt referral to specialists, as interventions such as corticosteroid or platelet-rich plasma injections, and ultrasound, have a varying degree of success in their effectiveness. Surgical intervention is primarily reserved for those who experience severe symptoms and have failed to respond to consistently performed nonoperative treatment over the course of several months.

Other causes of heel pain should also be considered. Calcaneus stress fracture presents differently, with more pain when a person is active, and less in the morning or with startup. Swelling may occur as well, and tenderness on examination is not limited to the plantar medial heel. A positive squeeze test of the calcaneus is pathognomonic for calcaneus stress fracture. Achilles tendinitis (covered later) should also be considered if the pain is more posterior.

Achilles Tendonitis

Achilles tendinopathy is secondary to overuse injury and is very common in athletes, especially those who run and jump. Patients typically will complain of pain over the Achilles tendon at its insertion point posteriorly and occasionally 6 to 10 cm above the insertion. Its pathology is accompanied by alterations in the tendon's structure and mechanical properties, altered lower extremity function, and fear of movement. These injuries acutely need to be treated with ice, NSAIDs, and reduction of activity. More involved treatment may be needed when symptoms persist and become chronic.[12]

Chronically, the pathology is not necessarily inflammatory but is rather a failed healing response. The pain could be related to the neurovascular ingrowth seen in the tendon's response to injury. MRI and ultrasound are helpful in confirming the diagnosis and guiding treatment.[13]

Initial treatments for the chronic symptoms are conservative, which may include NSAIDs, physical therapy, bracing, heel lifts, and footwear modification. Occasionally, complete rest and immobilization in a cast boot are necessary. If failed over a 6-month period of time, then the primary care provider may need to refer to an orthopedic specialist for further treatment up to and including surgery.[14]

PREVENTION OF INJURY

Reducing the frequency of injuries is important to keep people active, especially in the age group in which pickleball has become so popular. There is no literature to provide sport-specific training or equipment recommendations at present for pickleball specifically,[15] so preventative measure recommendations are based on the types of injuries that present. Prevention tactics for acute injuries include strength and endurance training, appropriate weight management, shoe orthoses, and appropriate-fitting shoes.[8] A proper pregame warm-up is also essential for prevention of both acute and chronic injuries.[15]

For prevention of chronic injuries, stretching the plantar fascia and calf before activity, garnering adequate rest, and not pushing beyond exertion are helpful.[12] The appropriate management of acute injuries is also imperative in the prevention of chronic issues.[13]

SUMMARY

With the substantial growth of the sport presently, familiarity with the most common presentations of injuries associated with participation in pickleball can help focus a differential list when patients present with acute or chronic injuries related to the sport.

A systematic review showed many benefits of participation in pickleball, including the fact that it is an inclusive sport that does not require adaptations. Participation in the sport is associated with significant improvements in personal well-being, life satisfaction, depression, stress, and happiness, among others.[16] Given these benefits, keeping patients participating is of importance, thus providing patients that participate in the sport with education regarding prevention of injuries and being knowledgeable in management of sustained injuries can serve to keep patients participating, and reaping the benefits, for a long time to come.

CLINICS CARE POINTS

- History: Inversion is the most common mechanism of injury in ankle sprains.[3]
- Physical examination: Comparing the injured and uninjured leg is essential.[10] Neurovascular evaluation is essential for all acute injuries.[6] There are special tests including:
  - Thompson's test for Achilles tendon rupture.[10]
  - Squeeze test of the calcaneus is pathognomonic for calcaneus stress fracture.[11]
- Ottawa ankle and foot rules are used to determine the necessity of ankle or foot x-rays.[6]
- The following should be referred to orthopedics, sports medicine, or another qualified specialist:
  - Patients with a suspected ankle sprain who fails the usual management[6]
  - Patients with a history of recurrent sprains and ankle instability[6]
  - A patient with a zone 2, zone 3, or dancer's fracture should be immediately referred.[9]
  - Suspected Achilles tendon rupture should immediately be referred.[10]
  - Patients with plantar fasciitis or Achilles tendonitis that fail initial/conservative treatments overtime[11,14]

DISCLOSURE

None.

REFERENCES

1. Mackie B. Pickleball statistics: America's fastest growing sport in 2023. Pickleheads. https://www.pickleheads.com/blog/pickleball-statistics. Published February 24, 2023. Accessed April 30, 2023.
2. Greiner N. Pickleball: Injury Considerations in an Increasingly Popular Sport. Mo Med 2019;116(6):488–91.
3. Changstrom B, McBride A, Khodaee M. Epidemiology of racket and paddle sports-related injuries treated in the United States Emergency Departments, 2007–2016. Physician Sportsmed 2021;50(3):197–204.
4. Biz C, Nicoletti P, Tomasin M, et al. Is Kinesio taping effective for sport performance and ankle function of athletes with chronic ankle instability (CAI)? A systematic review and meta-analysis. Medicina 2022;58(5):620.
5. Forrester MB. Pickleball-related injuries treated in emergency departments. J Emerg Med 2019;58(2):275–9.
6. Wolfe MW, Uhl TL, Mattacola CG, et al. Management of ankle sprains [published correction appears in Am Fam Physician 2001;64(3):386]. Am Fam Physician 2001;63(1):93–104.
7. Caldemeyer LE, Brown SM, Mulcahey MK. Neuromuscular training for the prevention of ankle sprains in female athletes: A systematic review. Physician Sportsmed 2020;48(4):363–9.

8. Attia AK, Taha T, Kong G, et al. Return to play and Fracture Union after the surgical management of jones fractures in athletes: A systematic review and meta-analysis. Am J Sports Med 2021;49(12):3422–36.
9. Anderson RB, Cohen BE. Stress Fractures of the Foot and Ankle. In: Coughlin M, Saltzman C, Anderson R, editors. Mann's surgery of the foot and ankle. 9th ed. Philadelphia: Elsevier Saunders; 2014. p. 1688–722.
10. Park S-H, Lee HS, Young KW, et al. Treatment of acute Achilles tendon rupture. Clinics in Orthopedic Surgery 2020;12(1):1.
11. Bourne M, Talkad A, Varacallo M. Anatomy, bony pelvis and lower limb, foot fascia. In: StatPearls. Treasure Island (FL): StatPearls Publishing; 2022.
12. Silbernagel KG, Hanlon S, Sprague A. Current clinical concepts: Conservative management of achilles tendinopathy. J Athl Train 2020;55(5):438–47.
13. Alfredson H, Cook J. A treatment algorithm for managing achilles tendinopathy: new treatment options. Br J Sports Med 2007;41(4):211–6.
14. Winfeld SB. Achilles Tendon Disorders. Med Clin 2014;98(2):331–8.
15. Vitale K, Liu S. Pickleball: Review and clinical recommendations for this fast-growing sport. Curr Sports Med Rep 2020;19(10):406–13.
16. Cerezuela J-L, Lirola M-J, Cangas AJ. Pickleball and mental health in adults: A systematic review. Front Psychol 2023;14. https://doi.org/10.3389/fpsyg.2023.1137047.

Orthopedic Emergencies
The Common and the Critical

Alan M. Keating, MPAS, PA-C*

KEYWORDS

- Orthopedic emergency • Musculoskeletal soft tissue injuries
- Critical acute fractures • Joint instability • Compartment syndrome
- Joint rehabilitation

KEY POINTS

- Emergent orthopedic medicine encompasses the treatment of simple soft tissue injuries to complex open fractures and compartment syndrome.
- The goals of acute orthopedic treatment are joint stability, pain reduction, injury repair, and improvement of function.
- Proper evaluation of acute orthopedic injuries will achieve these goals and avoid future chronic pain and deformities.
- Orthopedic treatment plans incorporate support or repair of the affected area, topical treatments, antiinflammatory medications, and physical therapy.

INTRODUCTION

Simply put, the human musculoskeletal system is a system of pulleys, hinges, and cables attached to a frame that moves our bodies from point A to point B. It also supports and protects our vital organ systems. However, it is a voluntary muscle system needing intentional neurostimulation to work. Acute orthopedic injuries cause defects in the structure, which reduce or prevent mobility. Appropriate orthopedic care involves detecting the damage and determining if it is structural, neurogenic, or both.

Identifying, acute fractures can be achieved with a simple 3-view plain film radiograph of the affected area. However, what happens if a complete evaluation with a thorough history gathering, physical examination, and subsequent additional imaging is not performed or not done efficiently? For example, a missed fracture of the scaphoid bone will leave the patient with years of pain and poor functioning. The most important responsibility of the nonorthopedic physician assistant is knowing how to assess, examine, and describe an acute injury to the patient and their

MPAS, University of Nebraska Medical Center
* 1553 Janmar Road, Snellville, GA 30078.
E-mail address: a-keating@att.net

Physician Assist Clin 9 (2024) 81–90
https://doi.org/10.1016/j.cpha.2023.07.009
2405-7991/24/© 2023 Elsevier Inc. All rights reserved.

orthopedic colleague. Knowing how to treat the injury, when to refer to orthopedics, and how best to describe the injury or fracture is imperative.

This article overviews the basic evaluation and treatment of the most common, and most importantly, critical orthopedic injuries.

FAST FACTS

- In 2020, 30% (38 million) of all emergency department visits (131 million) were for an injury.[1]
- It has been estimated that 20% of all emergency department visits are musculo-skeletal, and most patients are treated and discharged.[2]
- In 2021 there were 62 million injury visits (all clinical settings) in the United States, resulting in 224,935 avoidable deaths.[3]

THE MOST COMMON

The most common outpatient orthopedic chief complaints are adult knee pain, sports injuries of all ages, shoulder pain, and adult hip pain. Adult knee pain is prevalent due to work, sports, and overuse injuries. It is also the most common joint for arthritis in older adults, with osteoarthritis (OA) affecting more than 32.5 million US adults.[4] However, the highest occurring acute injuries are sprains and strains, tendon tears, dislocations, and fractures. Specifically, ankle/foot sprains, meniscus tears of the knee, rotator cuff tendon tears, anterior cruciate ligament (ACL) tears of the knee, wrist fractures, and shoulder dislocations occur most often. One study of US emergency departments noted that fractures alone account for about 60% of emergency room visits.[2] Overuse and chronic inflammatory disorders such as carpal tunnel syndrome, lateral epicondylitis, and plantar fasciitis are also commonplace.

STRAINS

Muscle strains occur when there is any tearing or stretching of the fascicles of muscle fibers. The large-speed muscles are the most frequently strained type of muscle. A high concentration of type II muscle fibers allows these muscles to contract quickly. They are found between 2 joints, usually large joints. The most common muscles to strain are the hamstring, gastrocnemius, and quadriceps. Strains frequently occur in athletes when they accelerate suddenly. The lumbar muscles also have a high frequency of straining, but it is more often due to heavy lifting or a fall.

The amount of damage to the muscle fibers categorizes strains. A grade I strain results in mild damage (less than 5% of fibers) with minimal loss of strength and motion. The recovery time will be in 2 to 3 weeks. A grade II strain creates moderate damage (20%–50%) with partial muscle rupture, significant loss of strength, and greater pain. The recovery can be 2 to 3 months. A grade III strain is a complete muscle or tendon rupture. There is often a palpable defect or deformity in the muscle, tendon, or tendon insertion site. Most large muscle strains are treated nonsurgically. It is important to stress to patients that incomplete rehabilitation of large muscle strains can result in reinjury, increased muscle damage, and reduced function.[5]

SPRAINS

Acute sprains occur with sudden stress on the stabilizing ligaments of large joints. The ligaments suffer stretching and tearing of structural fibers. Sprains are categorized by the degree of tearing of the ligaments and instability of the joint. A grade I sprain is a stable joint and will have minor to mild damage. The injury recovery time is about 2 to

3 weeks. A grade II sprain causes partial ligament tearing and may involve multiple ligaments. A grade II is stable, but recovery time can be 6 to 8 weeks. A grade III sprain is a complete ligament tear at the midportion or from its boney attachment. It is an unstable joint and often requires surgical repair.[6]

The ankle is the most common joint to sprain. Acute ankle sprains are either inversion (inward foot torsion) or eversion (outward foot torsion). Inversion sprains are due to lateral stress and occur more often than eversion (medial) sprains. Fortunately, most ankle sprains are mild (first- or second-degree). However, in the case of first-time grade I and II sprains, physical therapy is critical to restoring joint functioning. Undertreating these "simple" sprains can damage ankle proprioception and stability.[6] Incomplete physical therapy will result in ligamental laxity, leading to repeat sprains and possible ligament rupture. It is essential to rehabilitate the patient's acute ankle sprain fully.

The second most common joint to sprain is the knee, specifically the medial collateral ligament (MCL), lateral collateral ligament, and the ACL. The ACL sprain/tear, although not as common as the MCL, is extremely painful and often results in an acute effusion. Needle aspiration will yield serosanguinous fluid. It is pathognomonic for an ACL tear. An ACL tear creates an unstable knee joint due to insufficient anterior stabilization. Treat it with a knee immobilizer, complete activity restriction, and an orthopedic referral for surgical evaluation.

TENDON TEARS

Acute tendon tears and ruptures will require surgical repair. The most significant tendon ruptures are the patellar/quadriceps and Achilles tendons. These patients will present to urgent care and emergency departments shortly after the injury. They often describe a sudden severe "knifelike" pain at the joint with immediate loss of function. Frequently the injury occurs with sport activity or heavy lifting/pushing.

The patient with a patellar/quadriceps tendon rupture loses knee function and cannot extend the lower extremity. A lateral knee radiograph will show a severe patellar malalignment. Immediate knee immobilization with crutches, no weightbearing, and an orthopedic evaluation for surgery is appropriate management.

Patients with an Achilles tendon tear will have a positive Thompson test (total lack of passive plantar flexion with squeezing of the calf muscle) on examination. The sensitivity of the Thompson test is 96% to 100% for diagnosing a complete Achilles tendon rupture, but data are limited.[7] Stabilize the ankle/foot joint with a posterior splint or pneumatic boot. A surgical evaluation must be made quickly. A delay in the repair can cause muscle atrophy, making surgical repair difficult and creating a longer rehabilitation time.

DISLOCATIONS

Dislocations cause a complete separation of the 2 bones that form a joint. Trauma is often the reason for the dislocation, but it can be recurrent in an unstable joint. Subluxation is the partial separation of the joint. Ligamental and boney injuries can also take place during the dislocation. Clinically significant fractures are found in about 25% of all dislocations.[8] Dislocations have a high complication risk in large joints due to neurovascular compromise. Reduce dislocations as rapidly as possible, especially when neurovascular compromise is present. Any joint dislocation will need reduction, immobilization (splint/brace), and orthopedic evaluation to assess joint stability and surgical need.

The most common joint to dislocate is the shoulder (50.6%), followed by fingers (10.1%), toes (7.6%), hip (7.3%), and elbow (6.5%).[8,9] Ninety-five percent of shoulder dislocations are anterior.[10] The patient usually has a history of a posterior or lateral fall. It is painful, and the patient will show minimal mobility of the extremity. Always assess distal neurovascular status. A radiograph confirms the diagnosis with the humeral head in an anterior position in relation to the glenoid process. Unfortunately, the risk of recurrent shoulder dislocations is high. However, it depends on the age at the initial dislocation. The rate of recurrent dislocation is 72% to 100% for patients younger than 20 years, 70% to 82% for those aged 20 to 30 years, and 14% to 22% if age is greater than 50 years.[11]

FRACTURES

A fracture is a break in the cortex of the bone. It occurs when a force against the bone is greater than the bone's strength.[12] It is almost always acute except for stress, compression, or pathologic fractures. Fractures destabilize the bone and associated joint and can also involve sprains, dislocations, and tendon injuries in more severe cases. Most, however, are simple, with 1 or 2 fragments.

FRACTURE ASSESSMENT GUIDELINES

When evaluating and assessing an acute fracture, a clinician can use the following mnemonics, *NOM* and *TOAD*, to review the history and describe the fracture when referring to an orthopedic clinician.

NOM

NOM stands for *Neurovascular* status, *Open* (or closed fracture), and *Mechanism* of injury (and any additional trauma). This mnemonic will help focus the history and physical examination of a fracture injury.

Neurovascular status is the most vital part of an assessment. Without delay, assess the distal pulses of the affected extremity. Restore circulation quickly via closed or open fracture reduction. Next, evaluate and document nerve function. Any nerve deficit that does not immediately respond to the reduction of the fracture will need to be monitored. Neurapraxia (nerve contusion) should resolve in 6 to 8 weeks, but axonotmesis (nerve tissue damage—usually due to a crush injury) can take months to years to resolve.[12] The greater the trauma, the higher the likelihood of damage, possibly permanent.

Open versus closed portion of NOM. A fracture is open if there is any skin disruption overlying the fracture, regardless of visualization of the fractured bone. It is best practice to assume it is open and provide intravenous (IV) and oral antibiotic coverage. Lacerations and puncture or bite (animal or human) wounds overlying joints are treated similarly, even if a fracture is absent on a radiograph.

Mechanism of injury describes precisely how the injury occurred. A simple ankle sprain while walking does not have the same risk severity as a fall from a roof or crush injury to the lower extremity with entrapment for several hours (high risk of compartment syndrome). All potential trauma areas must be assessed, documented, and ruled out.

TOAD

The TOAD mnemonic is used when describing the fracture to an orthopedic provider (phone consult) or the patient/family.

What *Type* of fracture is present? Is it a simple fracture (transverse, avulsion, buckle, greenstick) or a complex fracture (spiral and comminuted) at several locations on the bone?

Open and closed status is the same as for the NOM pneumonic but needs to be included in the description.

Angulation is the degree of angulation of the distal bone fragment in relation to the proximal portion. Document in terms of measured degrees, such as "there are 25° of dorsal angulation." The greater the angulation, the greater need for reduction.

Displacement describes how much shifting occurs between the 2 fragments in any given plane (anterior/posterior, medial/lateral, dorsal/volar). It is reported in percentage, such as "there is a 50% lateral displacement of the distal radius." Displacement can occur in more than one plane. Long bone fractures are prone to significant displacement due to the contraction of the large muscles.

MISSED FRACTURES

Correctly treating an obvious fracture provides the best chance of proper healing and outcome. However, a missed fracture can lead to misdiagnosis, improper treatment, pain, malfunction, and deformity. It is better to assume the presence of a fracture even if not on radiograph. Fractures of the metatarsals, calcaneus, tibial plateau, scaphoid, radial head, cervical spine, and growth plates in children have a high false-negative rate on plain film radiograph.[13,14] Always treat pain in these areas with splinting, patient education, and referral to orthopedics for follow-up.

Two fractures that are important to not miss are cervical spine and scaphoid fractures. Cervical spinal pain should be evaluated with the *PANDA* mnemonic (**Table 1**). If any of these 5 points is positive on examination and documentation, then a plain film radiograph is required. The patient must be placed in a hard collar until cleared by radiology. The lateral view on cervical plain film radiograph is the most important. Nearly half of all cervical spine injuries affect C6 and C7.[15] If available, a computed tomography (CT) of the cervical spine is best. If the patient is older than 60 years or has significant osteoarthritic changes, CT is the only imaging that can definitively rule out an acute fracture.

Scaphoid fractures make up 60% to 70% of all carpal fractures and are missed as much as 40% on first presentation.[14] If there is "Snuff Box" tenderness (tenderness over the scaphoid—just distal to the medial-distal radius) on the examination then a scaphoid view is required. This view is an additional view in most facilities. Treatment is a thumb spica splint and orthopedic referral. Emphasize that follow-up orthopedic evaluation is essential. A delay in diagnosing a scaphoid fracture can lead to avascular necrosis, malunion, and nonunion.[16] Displaced scaphoid fractures have a high surgical repair rate.

Table 1 PANDA criteria	
P Pain	The patient describes pain or there is pain on palpation
A Alcohol	The patient has recently ingested alcohol
N Nerve Deficit	The presence of dramatic and painful injuries that distract from the neck assessment. This can occur in severe trauma.
D Distracting Injury	The presence of dramatic and painful injuries that distract from the neck assessment. This can occur in severe trauma.
A Altered Mental Status	Any mental status change on history or examination, even if only briefly

THE MOST CRITICAL

Emergent orthopedic injuries are often due to severe trauma such as motor vehicle collisions, high-level falls, assaults, and entrapment/crush injuries. Rapid assessment, diagnosis, and treatment are critical to limb survival and preventing severe complications. Large bone fractures, open fractures, and compartment syndrome are the most severe orthopedic emergencies, which always require immediate assessment, stabilization, treatment, and surgical intervention.

LARGE BONE FRACTURES

Large bone fractures (humerus, femur, tibia) are associated with higher angulation, displacement, and neurovascular injury rates. There will also be more edema from marrow and large vessel bleeding, with an increased risk of vascular compromise, but rarely enough to cause hemorrhagic shock. Posteriorly displaced supracondylar humeral fractures have a high risk of vascular compromise.[12] Large bone fractures must be quickly stabilized with splinting or traction. Most femur and tibial shaft fractures require surgical open reduction with internal/external fixation (ORIF). It is less often that humeral shaft fractures will need surgery but will need to be followed-up closely.

There are 2 additional complications with large bone fractures. The first is pulmonary embolism (PE), which is a high risk with hip or pelvic fracture fractures. PE is the most common fatal complication of significant hip or pelvis fractures. The second complication, a fat embolism, is more common in femoral fractures. Fat cells and other marrow contents may be released, creating emboli that travel to the lungs.[12]

OPEN FRACTURES

Skin disruption of any amount overlying a fracture is considered an open fracture. The most significant complication with open fractures is the high risk of infection, initially and for the first several weeks postoperatively. Infection risk is increased with contaminated and significantly displaced fractures, especially when the fractured bone is exposed. First and foremost, assess the neurovascular status distal to the fracture. Make sure to always radiograph the joints above and below the fracture. For example, an open (or closed) distal tibia fracture often results in fractures of the proximal tibia and/or femur. The fracture needs to be immediately reduced if compromise is present.

Per the 2015 American College of Surgeons Trauma Quality Improvement Program recommendations, IV antibiotics should be started within 60 minutes of hospital presentation, along with tetanus vaccination status verification.[17] The antibiotic to be initiated depends on the severity of the fracture and contamination, but a first-generation cephalosporin is recommended.[18] Aminoglycosides are recommended in more severe fractures, and penicillin is added if there is potential fecal or clostridial contamination.[19] Cover the wound with sterile saline-soaked gauze and splint, and consult an on-call orthopedist. Open fractures with irreducible joints and exposed articular cartilage require timely surgical management. Previously, that time has traditionally been within 6 hours of hospital arrival. New research supports no increase in infectious complications if the patient has surgical irrigation and debridement, within 24 hours.[20] Regardless of the operating room timing, surgical debridement and high-volume irrigation with ORIF will be required. Post-op antibiotic therapy is to be continued to reduce post-op infection risk.

COMPARTMENT SYNDROME

Compartment syndrome happens more often with fractures of the long bones. Roughly 75% of compartment syndrome cases are due to fractures of the tibia or radius.[21] Tissue edema occurs, secondary to bleeding, due to the fracture or crush injury. If the bleeding is not stopped, edema can develop within a closed fascial compartment (anterior or posterior compartments of the leg), and interstitial compartment pressure increases. Compartment syndrome can occur any time after the capillary pressure exceeds 8 mm Hg. It decreases cellular perfusion, creates an internal "tourniquet," and suppresses distal blood flow. Unfortunately, cellular perfusion can cease before distal pulses become undetectable. The resulting tissue ischemia creates further resistance, and the symptoms worsen.[22] It is recommended that diagnosis is made when the difference between the diastolic blood pressure and the compartment pressure (delta pressure) is 30 mm Hg or less.[23]

Compartment syndrome can also be seen in soft tissue crush injuries (without fracture), burns, tight bandaging, and casting. It can occur in the upper arm, abdomen, and buttocks. It can develop within hours or days. The primary symptoms are severe pain, edema, pallor, reduced distal pulses, and cyanosis.[22] Assess and describe any of these symptoms when evaluating a distal extremity fracture or crush injury. Place the affected limb level with the heart to prevent hypoperfusion.[24] Immediately consult orthopedics on-call. Early fasciotomy (ideally within 6 hours of symptom onset) can save the extremity.[24] It is performed to prevent complete necrosis, infection, and amputation.

OUTPATIENT ORTHOPEDIC TREATMENT PLAN

Musculoskeletal complaints comprise about 20% of primary care and emergency department visits annually in the United States.[25] The first encounter involves assessment, radiographs, and diagnosis. The initial treatment plan uses the basic mnemonic of RICE (Rest, Ice, Compression, and Elevation) for the first few days. However, recent research supports the notion that ice and rest may not enhance recovery.[26,27]

The DHAT mnemonic was taught to me 20 years ago by Dr Jimmy Spivey, who practiced orthopedic medicine for more than 50 years. This plan is effective for most injuries and disorders with few modifications. It can be given to the patient at the end of the visit.

DHAT

The DHAT treatment plan has 4 components: stabilize/support, localized thermal treatment, antiinflammatory medications, and therapy.

D stands for Don't make it worse. The patient will modify or decrease activity. Work or school restrictions are provided and modified at follow-up visits. The clinician should provide splints, casts, braces, crutches, and walkers for acute injuries. Overuse injuries or chronic pain areas are supported with removable bracing. Finally, surgery (stabilization) is performed to reduce and fix it into the proper position either externally (plaster and fiberglass casting) or internally (hardware).

H stands for Heat application over the area of injury after using ice. Intermittent (30–45 minutes and off for 2–3 hours) ice topically is appropriate for the first 2 to 3 days. However, once the patient can begin at-home therapy, heat (low-setting heating pad, warm/wet compress, gel pack) is applied for around 30 minutes 3 to 4 times daily.

A stands for Antiinflammatory drugs: several over-the-counter (OTC) topical nonsteroid antiinflammatory drugs (NSAIDs) can be applied to the affected area after the use of a heated compress. The patient may also take an OTC oral NSAIDs. Prescribe oral NSAIDs or steroids in more severe cases. However, first review with the patient the contraindications of NSAIDs (eg, history of or current gastrointestinal bleeds or surgery, hypertension, renal failure).

T stands for *Therapy*. Based on their injury, the patient is given a basic at-home provider-guided physical therapy treatment plan. Daily home therapeutic exercises are readily available online. The goal is for the patient to perform the exercises twice daily. Finally, office-based physical therapy is the best choice to maximize the chance of complete healing of orthopedic injuries. The protocol is usually 2 to 3 times weekly for 6 to 8 weeks, depending on the injury.

All orthopedic injuries create pain. It varies greatly depending on the injury severity, type, pain tolerance, and patient age. For example, children often tolerate fractures better than adults due to the increased flexibility of developing bones. However, only in the case of severe fractures or postoperative care are controlled substances for pain indicated or advised. They are only to be prescribed for short durations, and always discuss with the patient the black box warnings of the chosen medication.

SUMMARY

Acute orthopedic injuries occur at all times of the day in all age groups and settings. They create severe pain and sometimes deformities. Rapid assessment, examination, and imaging are required for accurate diagnosis. Basic emergent treatment requires stabilization, pain control, and orthopedic consult. Most orthopedic injuries do not need an immediate orthopedic consult or surgery but will require an orthopedic follow-up visit. The challenge for the nonorthopedic clinician is knowing when a consult is necessary.

CLINICS CARE POINTS

- Use the same assessment method for every fracture injury, whether simple or complex.
- Emergent orthopedic care involves stabilization, pain control, surgical consults, and antibiotics when appropriate.
- Use NOM and TOAD to assess and describe fractures effectively.
- If there is a possibility of fracture, assume there is one.
- Educate your patient and their family members.
- Simple soft tissue injuries can be successfully treated in the primary setting with the DHAT treatment plan.

DISCLOSURE

There is no financial relationship with any commercial interest related to the content of the article. This article was solely researched and developed by the author. The author has nothing to disclose.

REFERENCES

1. Cairns C, Kang K. National hospital ambulatory medical care survey: 2020 emergency department summary tables. Hyattsville, MD: National Center for Health Statistics; 2020.

2. Silverman ARC, Broome JN, Jarvis RC 3rd, et al. Using Emergency Department Data to Inform Specialty Strategy: Analyzing the Distribution of 13,777 Consecutive Immediate Orthopaedic Consults in an Urban Community Emergency Department. J Am Acad Orthop Surg Glob Res Rev 2020;4(2):e20.00005. https://doi.org/10.5435/JAAOSGlobal-D-20-00005.

3. National Safety Council. Injury Facts. Available at: https://injuryfacts.nsc.org/. Accessed at 27 April 2023.

4. CDC. Osteoarthritis. July 27, 2020. Available at: https://www.cdc.gov/arthritis/basics/osteoarthritis.htm. Accessed at 26 April 2023.

5. Campagne D. Overview of sprains and other soft-tissue injuries. Merck Manual Online; 2021. Available at. https://www.merckmanuals.com. Accessed at 29 April 2023.

6. Campagne D. Ankle sprain. Merck Manual Online; 2021. Available at. https://www.merckmanuals.com. Accessed at 21 April 2023.

7. Maffulli N. The clinical diagnosis of subcutaneous tear of the Achilles tendon. Am J Sports Med 1998;26(2):266–70.

8. Abrams R, Akbarnia H. Shoulder dislocation overview. National Institute of Health: National Library of Medicine; 2022. Available at. https://www.ncbi.nlm.nih.gov/books/NBK459125/. Accessed at 25 April 2023.

9. Nabian MH, Zadegan SA, Zanjani LO, Mehrpour SR. Epidemiology of Joint Dislocations and Ligamentous/Tendinous Injuries among 2,700 Patients: Five-year Trend of a Tertiary Center in Iran. Arch Bone Jt Surg 2017;5(6):426–34.

10. Campagne D. Shoulder Dislocations. Merck Manual Online; 2021. Available at. https://www.merckmanuals.com. Accessed at 26 April 2023.

11. Polyzois I, Dattani R, Gupta R, et al. Traumatic First Time Shoulder Dislocation: Surgery vs Non-Operative Treatment. Arch Bone Jt Surg 2016;4(2):104–8.

12. Campagne D. Overview of fractures. Merck Manual Online; 2021. Available at. https://www.merckmanuals.com. Accessed at 22 April 2023.

13. Miele V, Galluzzo M, Trinci M. Missed fractures in the emergency department, errors in radiology. Rome, Italy: Springer-Verlag Milan; 2012. p. 39–50.

14. Pinto A, et al. Errors in imaging patients in the emergency setting. Br J Radiol 2016;89(1061).

15. Berritto D, Pinto A, Michelin P, et al. Trauma Imaging of the Acute Cervical Spine. Semin Muscoskel Radiol 2017;21:184–98.

16. Gelberman RH, Wolock BS, Siegel DB. Fractures and non-unions of the carpal scaphoid. Journal of Bone Joint Surgury American 1989;71:1560–5.

17. American College of Surgeons Trauma Quality Improvement Program. Best Practice Manage Orthopedic Trauma. 2015;1–38. Available at https://www.facs.org/media/mkbnhqtw/ortho_guidelines.pdf. Accessed at 27 April 2023.

18. Hoff WS, Bonadies JA, Cachecho R, et al. East practice management guidelines work group: update to practice management guidelines for prophylactic antibiotic use in open fractures. J Trauma 2011;70:751–4.

19. Carver DC, Kuehn SB, Weinlein JC. Role of systemic and local antibiotics in the treatment of open fractures. Orthop Clin North Am 2017;48:137–53.

20. Srour M, Inaba K, Okoye O, et al. Prospective evaluation of treatment of open fractures: effect of time to irrigation and debridement. JAMA Surgery 2015;150:332–6.

21. Elliott KG, Johnstone AJ. Diagnosing acute compartment syndrome. Journal of Bone and Joint Surgery, British Volume 2003;85(5):625.

22. Campagne D. Compartment syndrome. Merck Manual Online; 2021. Available at. https://www.merckmanuals.com. Accessed at 29 April 2023.

23. McQueen MM, Court-Brown CM. Compartment monitoring in tibial fractures. The pressure threshold for decompression. Journal of Bone and Joint Surgery, British Volume 1996;78(1):99.
24. Torlincasi AM, Lopez RA, Waseem M. Acute compartment syndrome. NIH National Library of Health; 2023. Available at. https://www.ncbi.nlm.nih.gov/books/NBK448124/. Accessed at 25 April 2023.
25. Hammerberg, EM et al. Acute compartment syndrome of the extremities. Up to Date. March 9, 2023. Available at https://www.uptodate.com/contents/acute-compartment-syndrome-of-the-extremities. Accessed at 29 April 2023.
26. Miller A. Evaluation of Common Musculoskeletal Injuries in the Urgent Setting. MedEdPORTAL 2016;12:10514. Available at. https://www.ncbi.nlm.nih.gov/pmc/articles/PMC6440529/. Accessed 29 April 2023.
27. Scialoia D, Swartzendruber AJ. The R.I.C.E Protocol is a MYTH: A Review and Recommendation. Sport J 2020;24.

What Is Eating Your Bones?
Primary Bone Cancers

Kerri Jack, MHS, PA-C

KEYWORDS

- Primary bone cancers • Sarcoma • Osteosarcoma • Chondrosarcoma
- Limb-sparing surgery • Neoadjuvant chemotherapy • Adjuvant chemotherapy
- Ewing sarcoma

KEY POINTS

- Early diagnosis and intervention are essential in patients presenting with signs and symptoms consistent with bone cancer.
- Bone cancer can either be primary, originating within the bone, or secondary, arising in an outside primary site and spreading to the bone.
- A multidisciplinary approach is essential in the treatment of primary bone cancers and includes surgery, chemotherapy, and radiation.
- There are several prognostic factors in primary bone cancer, which include tumor grade, histology, staging, location of tumor, and presence of metastasis.

INTRODUCTION

Bone cancers can be classified as primary or secondary. Primary bone cancers arise from the bone itself and are rare cancers making up about 0.2% of all malignancies.[1] Osteosarcoma, chondrosarcoma, and Ewing sarcoma (ES) are examples of primary bone cancers. Less common primary bone cancers include undifferentiated pleomorphic cancer (formerly termed malignant fibrous histiocytoma), fibrosarcoma, chordoma, and giant cell tumor, which account for fewer than 5% of all primary malignant bone tumors.[2] Although primary bone cancers are rare, they are associated with significant morbidity and mortality, making early diagnosis and treatment essential. Treatment of primary bone cancers involves a multidisciplinary approach, which includes surgery, radiation, chemotherapy, or immunotherapy.

INCIDENCE

According to the Surveillance, Epidemiology, and End Results (SEER) program, it is estimated that there will be approximately 3970 new cases of all bone and joint cancer

Chatham University MPAS Program, Woodland Road, Pittsburgh, PA 15232, USA
E-mail address: k.jack@chatham.edu

Physician Assist Clin 9 (2024) 91–107
https://doi.org/10.1016/j.cpha.2023.07.010
2405-7991/24/© 2023 Elsevier Inc. All rights reserved.

physicianassistant.theclinics.com

diagnosed in 2023.[1,3] From 2016 to 2020, 24% of bone and joint cancer cases were in patients less than 20 years of age followed by 20- to 34-year-old age group, 55 to 64 year old, and 65 to 74 year old, respectively.[1] The median age of diagnosis is typically around 46 year old.[1] Although younger patients are more likely to be diagnosed, the highest percentage of deaths occurs in ages 65 to 74 years followed by those aged 75 to 80 year old.[1] The SEER program cancer statistics on bone and joint cancer states that the median age of death is 66 year old with a 5-year relative survival of 68.9%.[1]

PATHOPHYSIOLOGY

Pathophysiology varies between the primary bone cancers. There are several factors that could contribute to the formation of bone cancers including, the initiation of malignant transformation from one or more oncogenic events initiated by genetic deviations such as mutations, deletions, and amplifications increasing proliferation rate or interfering with cell differentiation.[3] Cell microenvironment must be favorable for cancer cells to grow which is a complicated process.[4] Understanding the bone microenvironment and the effects of cancer cells on this environment can help not only in understanding the development of bone cancers but may also help with development of potential targeted agents in the treatment of bone cancers.[4]

History and Physical Examination

A thorough history and focused musculoskeletal physical examination is important when assessing a patient with a suspected bone tumor (**Tables 1** and **2**).

DIAGNOSTIC STUDIES

Based on the history and physical examination, if one suspects a potential malignant tumor, diagnosis is based on radiologic studies, laboratory tests, and tissue biopsy. An initial plain film, lateral and anteroposterior views, is ordered to visualize the affected bone and to confirm suspicion. Each cancer has specific characteristics on x-rays, and though not diagnostic, it may give an indication to the type of cancer (**Box 1**). If plain radiographs show potential cancer, then further imaging, such as MRI, CT scan, bone scan, and potentially a PET scan, is needed to delineate the extent of the cancer and rule out metastatic disease. MRI is the gold standard to assess the extent of the tumor into surrounding soft tissue as well as neurovascular structures to determine staging.[9] When ordering an MRI, it should include one joint above and one joint below the location of the actual tumor to evaluate for "skip lesions" which occur mostly in high grade sarcomas and are associated with poor prognosis.[9] CT scans are typically ordered to help with identifying metastasis, especially in the lungs. CT scans in conjunction with PET scans are being ordered more often in cases of high-grade sarcoma to evaluate for metastasis but does not seem to be as effective in low or intermediate grade sarcomas given that they do not tend to uptake isotope, unlike the high-grade sarcomas.[5]

Histologic evaluation of the tumor is necessary to determine the grade and for final diagnosis to help aid in treatment. This is accomplished by a core needle biopsy or open excisional surgical biopsy. It may be necessary to involve interventional radiology depending on the location of the tumor along with an experienced oncologic surgeon to ensure the correct procedure is being performed. It is important for whomever is performing the biopsy to pay attention to where the incision is placed so that the biopsy tract is located in the potential surgical field as to not compromise potential future limb-sparing surgery.[9,27] Once biopsy is obtained, the specimen is sent for

Table 1
Presenting symptoms, history, and physical examination in patients with suspected primary bone cancer[5-10]

Presenting Symptoms	History	Physical Examination
Localized pain can be progressive and insidious	Any recent injuries?	Inspection to assess for warmth, skin color, and swelling of affected area.
Swelling	Any precipitating factors?	Palpation assessing for a mass or lump as well as tenderness/pain, size of mass, mobility, location, and firmness.
Limited range of motion	Duration of pain typically days to months as compared with years with benign conditions	Range of motion of affected joint/bone.
Pain worse at night	Family or personal history of cancer and genetic conditions	Assess neurovascular states of affected extremity.
Acute onset of pain may indicate pathologic fracture, although a rare finding.	Any systemic symptoms: fever, weight loss, malaise, night sweats	Palpation lymph nodes, liver, and spleen to assess for enlargement to rule out metastasis.

***Always assess the joint/bone above and below the affected area.

histologic evaluation and special studies to include immunohistochemistry, cytogenetics, flow cytometry, and electron microscopy which can all aid in the diagnosis as well as potential treatment options.

STAGING

Once the diagnosis is determined, staging of the tumor is essential in guiding treatment as well as prognosis. There are two staging systems used: American Joint Commission on Cancer (AJCC), also known as Tumor, Nodes, Metastasis (TNM) staging and the Musculoskeletal Tumor Society System (Surgical Staging or Enneking System). The AJCC system uses grade, size, and extent of tumor, nodal involvement, and metastasis, whereas the Enneking system uses surgical grade, local extent (extra- or intracompartmental), and metastasis.[11,12,28]

TREATMENT

Bone cancer treatment is a multidisciplinary approach and involves several specialists, including surgical oncology, medical oncology, and radiation oncology. Specific treatment will depend on a variety of factors including histologic type of cancer, location, extent, grade, and presence of metastasis. Treatment options include surgery, particularly limb salvage surgery, chemotherapy (neoadjuvant, before surgery, or adjuvant, after surgery), and radiation. Staging helps to determine if single treatment versus multimodal treatment is indicated. Mutational analyses are also being studied across all primary bone cancers to determine if there are targets that can be developed for future treatment.

It is important to consider the patient population, such as adolescents and young adults, when treating with chemotherapy and radiation. Both treatments can affect

Table 2
Comparison of primary bone cancers[3,5,11-25]

	Osteosarcoma	Chondrosarcoma	Ewing Sarcoma
Incidence	• Children/adolescent aged 10–19 y • Age >65 y	• Age 40–75 y ○ Median age 51 y	• Children/adolescent aged 10–19 y • Peaks age 15 y

Risk factors/etiology	• Paget's disease
	• Radiation
	• Radium for ankylosing spondylitis
	• Germline mutations
	  ○ Li-Fraumeni
	  ○ Retinoblastoma
		• Benign enchondroma or osteochondroma	• Chromosomal translocation
			  ○ EWS-FI1 oncogenic gene fusion

Most common sites affected	• Distal femur • Proximal tibia/humerus • Pelvis • Skull • Jaw bones	• Axial skeleton: pelvis, ribs, scapula, vertebrae • Proximal long bone: humerus, tibia	• Pelvis • Proximal long bones: femur, tibia, humerus • Scapula • Vertebrae
X-ray findings	• Moth-eaten • Sunburst appearance • Codman triangle • Soft tissue extension	• Mixed lytic/blastic activity • Rings and arcs • Endosteal scalloping.	• Moth-eaten • Codman triangle • "Onion peel" • Soft tissue extension
Treatment	Based on grade • Surgery • Neoadjuvant • Adjuvant chemotherapy	Based on grade/classification • Conventional/clear cell/high-grade: surgery • High grade dedifferentiated: consider same as osteosarcoma. • Mesenchymal:same as Ewing sarcoma • Radiation if not amenable to surgery or positive margins	• Neoadjuvant chemotherapy • Surgery • Adjuvant chemotherapy. • Radiation if not amenable to surgery

> **Box 1**
> **Radiographic characteristics seen on x-ray in primary bone cancers[6,8,9,26]**
>
> - Moth-eaten appearance—bone destruction with ragged edges due to multiple lytic lesions.
> - Permeative appearance—trabeculae are not completely destroyed.
> - "Onion skin or peel"—layers of partially formed and partially calcified bone.
> - Sunburst appearance—spiculated periosteal reaction
> - Codman's triangle—a cuff of periosteal new bone formation at the margin of the soft tissue mass
> - "Rings and arcs"—describes calcification pattern, rings represent sclerosis, and arcs represent chondroid matrix.
> - Osteolytic
> - Osteoblastic
> - Mixed

reproductive status. Providers need to have a discussion regarding infertility with the patient and family and refer to an infertility clinic for further information.

OSTEOSARCOMA
Introduction/Incidence

There are approximately 1000 new cases of osteosarcoma diagnosed each year in the United States. About 50% of these cases are in children and adolescents. The peak incidence occurs in the 10 to 19 years of age range, particularly around puberty. There is a second smaller peak in elderly patients greater than 65 years of age.[3,11]

Males have a 1.5 to 2 times higher incidence of osteosarcoma than women.[29] Osteosarcomas typically form in the metaphysis of the lower long bones, distal femur, proximal tibia, and proximal humerus.[14,15] Other locations include the pelvis, skull, and/or jaw bones, though these locations make up a small percentage.[16] In older individuals, the location of osteosarcoma is more variable but still typical in long bones.[15] At the time of diagnosis, 15% to 32% of patient will already have metastatic disease, the most common sites being the lung and skeleton.[16]

Etiology/Risk Factors

Osteosarcomas are believed to develop from mesenchymal stem cells during their differentiation into osteoblasts, chondrocytes, and adipocytes.[30] The differentiation process is complex but ultimately mesenchymal stem cells form into pre-osteoblasts, then osteoblasts, and eventually osteocytes because of mutational changes as well as exposure to the surrounding microenvironment. When there is a change in the environment or an effect on mutation, cancer cells can develop instead of the typical cell lineage you would see in bone formation, repair, or stabilization.[30]

Most cases of osteosarcoma are sporadic, but in elderly patients, it is more commonly associated with Paget's disease, prior radiation therapy in those who had Hodgkin disease, and in those who received radium for ankylosing spondylitis.[12,14,15] Paget's disease is a metabolic disorder which causes exaggerated bone remodeling due to abnormal osteoclast regulation which shows that osteosarcoma formation may be related to bone remodeling.[16] Osteosarcoma has also been seen with germline mutation disorders such as Li-Fraumeni syndrome (p53 oncogene) and retinoblastoma (Rb oncogene alteration) as well as less common disorders such as Rothmund-Thomson syndrome, Bloom syndrome, and others.[12,15,17] Germline mutations affect the mesenchymal stem cell differentiation, whereas sporadic mutations affect the pre-osteoblast differentiation.[30]

There has been some discussion regarding the association between hormonal changes during puberty and the development of osteosarcoma. Insulin-like growth factor and other hormones are elevated during puberty which can be linked to carcinogenesis.[14] Being that the growth plate is found in the metaphysis of the long bone where there is rapid growth, especially in the adolescent ages, this shows a potential relationship between rapid bone growth and formation in the development of osteosarcoma.[11,18] Birth weight and height have also been under investigation for potentially contributing to the risk of osteosarcoma as well as chromosomal abnormalities.[14]

Classification of Osteosarcoma

Osteosarcomas are classified as primary, based on location, or secondary due to Paget's or radiation.[16] Location of osteosarcoma can include central or intramedullary, cortical, or surface.[16] Conventional, or classic, sarcoma is intramedullary and makes up about 85% of all osteosarcomas and is considered high grade, meaning that the cells are more abnormal and tend to grow or spread more rapidly.[16,18] Conventional osteosarcomas are further subdivided based on cell type, osteoblastic, fibroblastic, and chondroblastic.[11,31,32] Other intramedullary osteosarcomas include small cell and telangiectasia.[16] Surface osteosarcomas include periosteal and paraosteal.[11,16] Osteoblastic is the most common subtype making up about 60% of cases, followed by equal incidence of fibroblastic and chondroblastic types, followed by the rare variant subtypes.[30]

Diagnostic Findings

The first diagnostic test in the workup of osteosarcoma is a plain radiograph. There are specific findings on plain x-rays that can help determine if a tumor is high grade versus low grade. In high-grade osteosarcoma, the tumor will have a destructive lesion that appears "moth-eaten" with poorly defined margins, sunburst appearance, Codman's triangle, and about 75% of osteosarcomas will show soft tissue extension.[29,16,18] Differentiation of subtypes may also be seen on plain radiographs. If the tumor is osteoblastic, it may be described as "cloud-like" showing a more sclerotic appearance.[16] In chondroblastic subtype, the x-ray description may state "arcs and rings" calcification signifying cartilaginous involvement and fibroblastic predominate lesions will have a more lytic appearance.[16] Once the diagnosis is confirmed, tissue confirmation, MRI, and computerized tomography (CT) scan are then completed to assess for metastasis as well as extent of tumor in preparation for potential surgical intervention.

Laboratory studies will not help in the diagnosis of osteosarcoma but will help in determining any underlying organ abnormalities to serve as a baseline or show a contraindication to surgery or chemotherapy. Typical laboratory studies ordered include a complete blood count (CBC) with differential, basic metabolic panel (BMP), and liver function tests (LFTs). There are two serum tumor markers, alkaline phosphatase (ALP) and lactate dehydrogenase (LDH) that can be useful in the evaluation of osteosarcoma.[12,30] ALP levels can be elevated by 40% normal value and seems to be most predictive of tumor volume and poorer prognosis.[30]

Biopsy is completed to confirm the diagnosis of osteosarcoma. Microscopically, there will be a lace-like pattern of osteoid deposition with pleomorphic mesenchymal cell (**Fig. 1**).[33] With any biopsy, staining for specific biomarkers are completed. Biomarkers such as SATB2 and osteocalcin have been found in osteoblastic

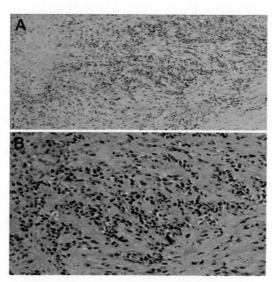

Fig. 1. Microscopic imaging of osteosarcoma.[33] Medium-power (*A*) and high-power (*B*) microscopic images of an osteosarcoma specimen, showing high cellularity, nuclear polymorphism, atypia, and disorganized osteoid production.

osteosarcomas but will not distinguish if the tumor is malignant or not.[30] Disorganized osteoid production, however, is a clinical hallmark of osteosarcoma.[33]

Treatment

The goal of treatment is to increase disease-free survival. High-grade osteosarcoma has a high risk of metastasis. At the time of diagnosis, about 80% to 90% of patients will already have distant metastasis either already visible on scans (10%–20%) or micrometastasis not yet visible, resulting in a poor prognosis.[11] Owing to the poor prognosis, standard treatment includes neoadjuvant chemotherapy, followed by surgical resection which is then followed by adjuvant chemotherapy.

Neoadjuvant chemotherapy is given before surgical resection, with a goal of eliminating micrometastasis, induces necrosis, and decreases the tumor size to increase feasibility of limb salvage surgery. Neoadjuvant chemotherapy helps to increase disease-free survival in patients. Response to chemotherapy is a prognostic factor.[17] Neoadjuvant chemotherapy is typically a multidrug regimen given IV for two cycles, consisting of cisplatin, doxorubicin (Adriamycin), methotrexate with leucovorin rescue, and ifosfamide with or without etoposide.[11,18]

Surgical resection consists of limb-sparing or amputation of the affected extremity depending on size of tumor, location, and tumor response after chemotherapy. Limb-sparing surgery is preferred and can be performed in 85% to 90% of patients diagnosed with osteosarcoma.[11] The goal of surgery is to remove the entire tumor and to obtain clear margins to decrease recurrence or metastasis. Limb-sparing surgery is to restore the function of bone and joint after resection and is performed in two steps: resection of the tumor and surrounding bone/soft tissue to obtain clear margins followed by reconstruction through endoprosthetic replacement or biological reconstruction such as allograft or autograft.[11,33,34,35] Amputation is another surgical intervention used if the limb is unable to be preserved, or complete resection with clear margins is not able to be achieved due to size or location of tumor or poor response to neoadjuvant chemotherapy.[33,19]

Adjuvant chemotherapy, that is, chemotherapy given after surgical intervention, is recommended to start within 21 days after surgery.[30,19] The goal of adjuvant chemotherapy is to decrease the incidence of any residual tumor cells. The same chemotherapy that was given preoperatively is typically given postoperatively for a total of six cycles (including the two cycles before surgery, providing a positive response was found with the initial treatment, meaning that tumor necrosis was >90%).[19] If a patient has a poor response after neoadjuvant chemotherapy, less than 90% necrosis, then one can consider changing the postoperative chemotherapy regimen.[12,19]

Osteosarcoma is typically radiotherapy resistant, so radiation is not a mainstay of treatment.[3] Although there have been studies showing that in patients who undergo surgical resection and negative margins are not able to be achieved, radiation may have a benefit as well as in areas that may be considered high risk for surgery.[3,11]

There are ongoing studies looking at several other treatment options for osteosarcoma, including immunotherapy, tyrosine kinase inhibitors, bone targeting therapies, DNA repair targeting, fusion protein targeting, and monoclonal antibodies.[12,30,33]

Metastatic/Recurrent Osteosarcoma

For those who present with metastatic disease on presentation, the first question is if the metastases can be resected or not. Depending on this, the treatment remains the same as for those who did not present with metastatic disease, neoadjuvant chemotherapy, surgery of both primary and metastatic disease, and follow with adjuvant chemotherapy.[34,35] Ifosfamide with or without etoposide is two chemotherapy regimens that can be used in recurrent or metastatic disease but comes with a higher toxicity profile.[33,35] There are several other second-line therapies available depending on what was received with initial treatment and include gemcitabine, docetaxel, sorafenib, or regorafenib.[2] If the metastatic disease is unable to be surgically resected, stereotactic radiation therapy, radiofrequency ablation, and cryotherapy can be considered.[2]

Prognosis

Prognosis of osteosarcoma depends on the histology of osteosarcoma, grade, location, and presence of metastasis.[33] Other prognostic factors include levels of C-reactive protein (CRP) and LDH, age, and response to neoadjuvant chemotherapy, amount of necrosis.[33] The 5-year survival rate for patients with localized disease is around 60%, whereas patients who develop recurrence, or present with metastasis at diagnosis, have a 5-year overall survival of less than 20%.[34] Patients who have a positive treatment response (tumor necrosis >90%) have a 5-year survival of 75% to 90% compared with those who do not have a positive response who have a 5-year survival of 45% to 60%.[8,34] Patients who develop local or distant recurrent disease greater than 2 years out from diagnosis have the potential for a 5-year survival rate of 45% providing the disease can be surgically resected.[33]

EWING SARCOMA
Introduction/Incidence

ES is estimated to occur in one in 100,000 in those 10 to 19 years of age with a peak incidence at age 15 years.[18] It accounts for 2% of childhood cancer and has a male-to-female ratio of 1.5 with worse prognosis in males.[3,5] The most common location of ES is the pelvis, followed by the proximal long bones such as the femur, tibia, humerus, and scapula but can also occur in flat bones as well.[5,7,13] In those patients that are diagnosed with ES, 20% will present with extraosseous tumors that can arise in any organ, more commonly in paravertebral and thoracic soft tissue.[7,36] Typical sites of metastatic involvement with ES include bone, bone marrow, and lung with about 20% to 25% presenting with metastasis at diagnosis.[3]

Etiology/Risk Factors

The etiology of ES is unknown, but it is thought that it is derived from undifferentiated, mesenchymal, or neuroectodermal cells and is part of the round cell family.[20] In ES, chromosomal translocation between TET and ETS genes is the molecular event leading to a reciprocal chromosomal translocation of FL11 gene on 11q24 and ESW gene 22q12, t(11;22) q24:q12, leading to ESW-FL11 oncogenic gene fusion which then acts as pathogenic transcription factor leading to tumor development.[20,37] There are several other translocations that can also contribute to the formation of ES but t(11;22) is the most common translocation occurring in about 85% to 90% of ES diagnoses.[20,38] The second most common translocation occurs on translocation t(21;12) (22;12) resulting in EWS-ERG fusion[13] occurring in about 10% to 15% of those with ES.[3,20] There are no other known risk factors in the development of ES such as environmental, familial cancers, or previous radiation.[37]

Classification

ES falls under the classification of round cell tumors. This class of tumors also includes Atkin's tumor and primitive neuroectodermal tumor (PNET) being that they share the same morphology and immunohistochemical features.[26] PNETs are less common than Ewing and make up only about 10% of the Ewing-like tumors.[5]

Diagnostic Findings

ES is diagnosed radiographically and histologically. The initial x-ray of the suspected area will show multiple confluent lytic lesions described as a "moth eaten" appearance, displaced periosteum (Codman's triangle), proliferative reaction described as "onion peel", and soft tissue extension.[7,26] With the pelvis being the most common site, these lesions are difficult to see on plain x-ray, so CT scan and MRI are a necessary part of the workup, to not only detect pelvic lesions but also help in staging the lesions by determining the extent of disease and evaluating for metastatic disease. Bone scans may also be used for determining bone metastasis as well as PET/CT scans, which do have higher sensitivity and specificity as compared with bone scan.[19] Bone marrow biopsy may be indicated if PET/CT scan shows bone metastasis.

Once radiographic imaging is completed, histologic diagnosis is imperative. A biopsy should be performed, and the collected tissue sent for evaluation. The main histologic finding is sheets of small, round, blue cells with a prominent nucleus and scant cytoplasm (Fig. 2).[26,20] Immunohistochemistry staining reveals expression of CD99 (MIC2) (Fig. 3), as well as CD56, vimentin, FLI1 (Fig. 4), HNK1, and CAV1.[3,26,20] If immunohistochemistry does not reveal CD99 expression, this rules out the diagnosis of ES. The other piece to diagnosing ES is completing in situ hybridization or rapid quantitative polymerase chain reaction to detect the chromosomal translocation t(11;22) (q24,q12) which is confirmatory for ES.[26,19,20]

Laboratory studies are nonconfirmatory in ES, although an elevated serum LDH has been shown to correlate to tumor burden and has a diagnostic and prognostic factor.[26] One may also see anemia and leukocytosis with ES as well as increases in erythrocyte sedimentation rate (ESR), ALP, and CRP, which can mimic an inflammatory response so clinicians will need to be careful when making a diagnosis.[7] Elevated

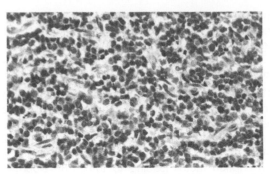

Fig. 2. Microscopic imaging in Ewing sarcoma.[20] ES/PNET composed of sheets of small round blue cells.

LDH is associated with a poorer prognosis as per a few studies that have been completed but other studies have not shown a correlation with prognosis.[36]

Treatment

ES is treated similarly to osteosarcoma with neoadjuvant chemotherapy, surgery, and adjuvant chemotherapy with the only difference in types of chemotherapy used and radiation available for patients whose cancer is not amenable to surgery.[7,17] Current cytotoxic medications that are used in ES include, doxorubicin, etoposide, cyclophosphamide, vincristine, dactinomycin, and ifosfamide, which are all given intravenously for about 12 weeks (6 cycles every 2 weeks) before reassessing for surgery.[19] The goal of neoadjuvant chemotherapy is to treat any potential micrometastatic disease and decrease tumor size to aid in surgical resection.

Local control includes limb salvage surgery and is determined based on location and size of tumor and if negative surgical margins can be achieved. Once neoadjuvant

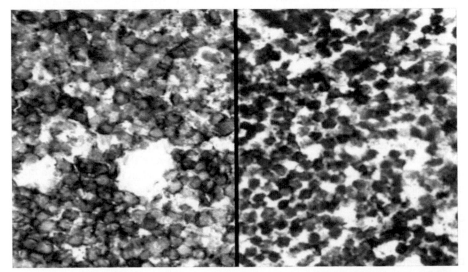

Fig. 3. Immunohistochemistry staining in Ewing family of tumors (EFT).[20] The tumor cells of EFT show membranous expression of CD99/MIC2 (*left*), and nuclear positivity for antibodies against FLI1 (*right*).

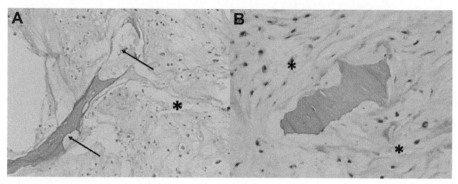

Fig. 4. Microscopic imaging of chondrosarcoma.[6] Microscopic images showing cartilaginous matrix-producing tumor (*asterisk*) with permeation into the bone [(*A*) H&E × 100; *arrow*] and entrapping the preexisting lamellar bone [(*B*) H&E × 200].

chemotherapy is completed, the same initial restaging scans are done to determine response rate based on the amount of necrosis present and if still amenable to surgery.[19] The goal of surgery is to completely resect the tumor while obtaining negative margins. If negative margins are unable to be obtained during surgery, then radiation therapy would be considered after surgery.[19] If the tumor is not in a location that is amenable to surgery, neoadjuvant chemotherapy is still given but would be followed by radiation therapy alone, rather than surgery.[19]

Definitive radiation therapy, without surgical resection, is associated with a higher risk of local recurrence but no effect on distant control.[21] Radiation should be considered postoperatively if there are positive surgical margins or if there has been an incomplete histologic response to neoadjuvant chemotherapy defined as greater than 10% viable tissue present on pathology.[2]

Metastatic/Recurrent Ewing Sarcoma

At the time of diagnosis, 20% to 25% of patients already have metastatic disease in the lung, bone, or bone marrow.[36] Chemotherapy in this setting is the treatment of choice, although in those patients who are found to have lung metastasis at the time of diagnosis, chemotherapy, surgery, and radiation can still be considered treatment options.[19] If a patient has disseminated metastatic or recurrent disease, it is recommended to consider treatment on clinical trial.

For those patients who undergo initial treatment, around 30% to 40% will still develop local or distant recurrence within 2 years of diagnosis.[19] For these patients who develop local recurrence, surgery or radiation can still be considered for treatment to obtain local control.[39] For distant recurrence, there are several factors to take into consideration as to what treatment options should be offered, including prognostic factors, such as timing of recurrence, site of recurrence, prior therapy, and patient characteristics such as any end-organ damage from previous treatment or other medical conditions and patient preference.[19,39] There are several chemotherapy options that have some effectiveness in metastatic or recurrent ES. Chemotherapy options include cyclophosphamide; topotecan, irinotecan, and temozolomide; etoposide single agent or combined with carboplatin or cisplatin; and gemcitabine with docetaxel.[13,19,39] When prescribing these chemotherapy regimens, practitioners need to make sure patients are aware that treatment of recurrent ES is not curative and also make them aware of the associated potential side effects, especially myelosuppression, and how each agent is administered in order for patients to make an informed decision on treatment choice.

Prognosis

There have been several prognostic factors in ES which include the presence of metastasis/stage of disease, primary tumor site, size, and response to therapy.[36] Patients with a primary tumor located in the axial skeleton, specifically the pelvis, are associated with a poorer survival than those with the primary tumor located in the diaphysis.[36] Large tumors greater than or equal to 8 cm or volume greater than or equal to 200 mL, and those who have had a poor histologic response to therapy, that is, less than 90% necrosis, are also associated with a poorer outcome.[36] The single most prognostic factor is disease-free interval from the time of diagnosis to first relapse.[39] Those who have first recurrence within 2 years of diagnosis, have a 5-year survival rate of 7% compared with those with first recurrence more than 2 years from diagnosis who have a 5-year survival rate of 30%.[39]

With advances in therapy, 5-year survival rate in ES patients who present with localized disease is 70%.[26] For those who develop recurrence or present with metastatic disease, the 5-year survival is less than 20%.[26] Patients with metastatic disease at diagnosis, the 5-year survival rate is 30% but if they present with metastasis in the lung only, the 5-year overall survival rate is 40%.[26,19] Bone and bone marrow metastases provide a lower long-term overall survival rate of 20%.[19]

CHONDROSARCOMA
Introduction/Incidence

Chondrosarcomas are slow growing tumors accounting for around 20% to 25% of all primary bone cancer and occurs in about 1 in 200,000 persons.[17] It is the most common bone cancer found in adults aged 40 to 75 years with a median age of 51 years.[3,17] Male to female incidence may deviate slightly toward males, but this varies by subtype.[22] Chondrosarcomas occurs primarily in the axial skeleton such as the pelvis, vertebrae, ribs and scapula, and proximal long bones such as humerus and tibia.[6,17,40] Medullary cavity of the metaphysis is the more typical location.[6] The risk of metastasis with chondrosarcoma varies with grade and subtype, but the lung is the most common site for metastasis and the incidence for lung metastasis in chondrosarcoma is 11.2%.[6,41]

Etiology/Risk Factors

Chondrosarcomas can develop from cartilage-producing chondrocyte cell, from a mesenchymal stem cell sporadically, or they can develop from benign enchondromas or osteochondromas.[2,17] Osteochondromas are benign cartilaginous lesions that develop on the surface of the bone, whereas enchondromas are benign lesions that develop in the medullary cavity of the bone.[42] The benign lesions transform into chondrosarcomas by the loss of specific proteins (EXT protein in osteochondromas) and mutations (isocitrate dehydrogenase [IDH] mutation in enchondroma), which are responsible for malignant transformation.[42] There are no other known risk factors in the development of chondrosarcomas.[17]

Classification

Chondrosarcomas are classified according to histologic characteristics and are considered low (Gr1), intermediate (Gr2), or high grade (Gr3).[3] Low-grade chondrosarcoma is also called atypical cartilaginous tumors (ACTs).[32]The most common subtype is conventional chondrosarcoma, accounting for 85% of all chondrosarcomas which can be further characterized into central, periosteal, or peripheral based on location in the bone.[6,22,24] Primary conventional chondrosarcoma arises independently of any risk factors and secondary chondrosarcoma arises from a preexiting condition.[22] Other subtypes include mesenchymal, clear cell, and dedifferentiated.[40,22]

Most conventional chondrosarcomas are low to intermediate grade and about 5% to 10% are high grade and most commonly occur in the central bone.[42,23] Central chondrosarcomas are typically secondary to enchondromas, whereas osteochondromas are precursors to the development of peripheral chondrosarcomas.[42] Secondary chondrosarcomas are typically low grade and can be seen in young adults aged 30 to 60 year old with a mean age of 34 years.[22] Periosteal chondrosarcomas occur in the periosteum and rarely arise on the surface of the bone, with occurrence seen more commonly in males in the third to fourth decade of life.[22]

Clear-cell chondrosarcomas are low-grade and are most likely to grow in the epiphysis of the long bones and tend to affect male patients more than females in their 30s to 50s.[22]

Mesenchymal chondrosarcomas are small round blue cell tumors that are high grade, which contributes to a higher risk of metastasis as well as involvement of the soft tissue.[22,43] They most commonly occur in the jaw then the ribs and spine, have a poorer prognosis, and develop in patients with a mean age of 25 year old.[22,43]

Dedifferentiated chondrosarcoma is a chondrosarcoma that occurs in 50 to 70 year olds and has transitioned from a conventional chondrosarcoma to a high grade, more aggressive cancer.[22] This histology type occurs in the same bone as conventional chondrosarcoma and this differentiation occurs in about 10% to 20% of patients with conventional type.[22] The dedifferentiation can occur peripherally or centrally. If a cartilage cap thickness of more than 2 cm is seen, this is suggestive of malignant transformation of osteochondroma to dedifferentiated chondrosarcoma.[23]

Diagnostics

As with osteosarcoma and ES, the initial workup of chondrosarcoma includes radiographic studies, followed by CT and/or MRI, and biopsy. Radiologic studies show calcified mixed lytic and blastic activity with "rings" and "arcs" along with endosteal scalloping which appears lobulated.[22] High-grade chondrosarcoma will show a moth-eaten appearance on x-ray.[22] MRI, with and without contrast, is the gold standard for diagnosing chondrosarcoma and will demonstrate low intensity on T1-weighted images and high intensity on T2-weighted images with potential post-enhancement.[22] CT scan will help with matrix mineralization as well as assess for extraosseous soft tissue extension.[22]

Histologic features seen on biopsy with chondrosarcoma include hyaline cartilage matrix, permeative pattern, increased cellularity, cellular atypia of chondrocytes, binucleated cells, entrapping of the preexisting of the lamellar bone, along with cellular changes (see **Fig. 4**).[6] Tumor grade under the microscope is based on cellularity, cellular/nuclear atypia, and mitoses.[6]

Treatment

Treatment is based on grade, location of tumor, patient factors, presence of metastasis, and tumor relationship to surrounding vital structures.[22] Chondrosarcoma, particularly conventional and clear cell, do not typically respond to chemotherapy or radiation because of slow growth of the tumor due to slow mitotic rate as well as decrease in vascularity of the tumor.[22] High-grade dedifferentiated chondrosarcoma is treated similarly to osteosarcoma and mesenchymal chondrosarcoma due to small cell component and may be treated with systemic chemotherapy similar to ES.[23,24]

Surgical resection with limb salvage procedures or amputation is the primary treatment for intermediate- or high-grade chondrosarcomas.[22,25] Low-grade/ACTs are typically treated with intralesional curettage resection followed by potential adjuvant application of liquid nitrogen followed by applying bone graft to the cavity made by resection.[22,25] If surgery is unable to obtain negative margins, then radiation therapy should be considered because positive margins are considered a risk factor for disease recurrence or metastasis.[22] Radiation can also be used if resection is not an option based on the location of the tumor or if the patient is not a surgical candidate due to other comorbidities.

New treatments are on the horizon looking at different pathways and mutations that could prove beneficial. A few areas that are being tested include IDH1 inhibitors, PIK3-AKT-mTOR inhibitors, cell cycle inhibitors, and epigenetic or immune modulators.[23,44]

Metastatic/Recurrent Chondrosarcoma

Chondrosarcomas that are unresectable or are high grade have an affinity for metastasis, especially to the lungs.[44] Sixty-five percent of patients with dedifferentiated or high-grade chondrosarcoma developed metastasis and 90% of all patients with dedifferentiated subtype develope pulmonary metastasis within 2 months of diagnosis.[41] Treatment of metastatic or recurrent disease has not been fully determined. If there is only local recurrence of the primary site, it is typically recommended to undergo surgical management as one would with initial diagnosis. If positive margins or tumor is unable to be surgically resected, then radiation therapy can be considered.[41] Patients presenting with oligometastatic disease of the lung could be considered for surgical resection as compared with those presenting with disseminated disease that may need systemic treatment.[24] Ultimately, a multidisciplinary approach to treatment in those with metastatic disease is necessary.

Prognosis

The biggest predictive prognostic factor for chondrosarcoma is histologic grade. Grade 1, atypical, or low grade has a 90% survival, grade 2 has a 5-year survival of around 75%, and grade 3 overall has a 5-year survival rate of 30%.[6,17,22] Dedifferentiated tumors have a 5-year survival rate of a 0% to 24% survival.[6] Other prognostic factors associated with survival include age, size of the lesion (>8 cm), location, whether the tumor is central or peripheral, and primary or secondary.[22,45] Secondary chondrosarcomas have a higher overall survival, with a 5-year survival rate around 90% as compared with primary chondrosarcoma.[6] Those who present with metastatic disease at diagnosis have a 5-year survival of 28%.[6]

SUMMARY

Primary bone cancers offer challenges to the clinician in not only the diagnosis but also treatment. Primary bone cancers are rare, but it is important to be suspicious in anyone presenting with localized pain, worse at night, with no underlying injury. It is important to obtain an appropriate history, physical examination, and diagnostics to aid in early diagnosis of primary bone cancer. Histologic confirmation will allow the clinician to engage a skilled multidisciplinary team to begin treatment consisting of surgery, chemotherapy, and possibly radiation, again based on the type of primary bone cancer. Treatment should be tailored to the patient based on other comorbidities, location and size of tumor, and if the cancer has metastasized or not. Long-term survival with primary bone cancer is possible if diagnosed early so it is imperative for clinicians to understand primary bone cancers.

CLINICS CARE POINTS

- Primary bone cancer is a rare cancer that arises from the bone itself that occurs in children, adolescents, and young adults with a suspicious presentation of progressive pain, worse at night, without underlying injury.

- Osteosarcoma and Ewing sarcoma most commonly occur in children and adolescents, whereas chondrosarcoma occurs in adults.

- Surgery, limb-sparing or amputation, is the mainstay treatment of all primary bone cancers and is an involved procedure that takes careful planning and discussions regarding the risks, complications, and potential long-term activity restrictions.

- Systemic chemotherapy is used in both osteosarcoma and Ewing sarcoma, but in chondrosarcoma, it is based on classification and can potentially be used in dedifferentiated and mesenchymal. Most chondrosarcomas are resistant to chemotherapy.

- Osteosarcomas are typically radioresistant, and radiation is not used as a primary treatment option. If the tumor is not amenable to surgery or margins are positive after surgery, radiation may be considered.

DISCLOSURE

The author has no financial or nonfinancial disclosures.

REFERENCES

1. National Cancer Institute Surveillance, Epidemiology, and End Results Program, Cancer Stat Facts: Bone and Joint Cancer. Available at: https://seer.cancer.gov/statfacts/html/bones.html. Accessed February 8, 2023.
2. Casali PG, Bielack S, Abecassis N, et al. Bone sarcomas: ESMO-PaedCan-EURACAN Clinical Practice Guidelines for diagnosis, treatment, and follow-up. Ann Oncol 2018;29(Suppl 4):iv79–95.
3. Brown HK, Schiavone K, Gouin F, et al. Biology of Bone Sarcomas and New Therapeutic Developments. Calcif Tissue Int 2018;102:174–95.
4. Bădilă AE, Rădulescu DM, Niculescu A-G, et al. Recent Advances in the Treatment of Bone Metastases and Primary Bone Tumors: An Up-to-Date Review. Cancers 2021;13(16):4229.
5. Bernthal NM, Burke ZC, Blumstein GW, et al. Musculoskeletal Oncology. In: McMahon PJ, Skinner HB, editors. Current Diagnosis & Treatment in Orthopedics, 6e. McGraw Hill; 2021. Available at: http://accessmedicine.mhmedical.com/content.aspx?bookid=3066&sectionid=2557233740. Accessed October 20, 2022.
6. Gazendam A, Popovic S, Parasu N, et al. Chondrosarcoma: A Clinical Review. J Clin Med 2023;12(7):2506.
7. Ozaki T. Diagnosis and treatment of Ewing sarcoma of the bone: a review article. J Orthop Sci 2015;20(2):250–63.
8. Isakoff MS, Bielack SS, Meltzer P, et al. Osteosarcoma: Current Treatment and a Collaborative Pathway to Success. J Clinical Oncol 2015;33(27):3029–35.
9. Plant J, Cannon S. Diagnostic work up and recognition of primary bone tumors: a review. EFORT Open Rev 2017;1(6):247–53.
10. Pullan JE, Lotfollahzadeh S. Primary Bone Cancer. In: StatPearls [Internet]. StatPearls Publishing; 2023. Available at: https://www.ncbi.nlm.nih.gov/books/NBK560830/. Accessed February 1,2023.

11. Zhao X, Wu Q, Gong X, et al. Osteosarcoma: A review of current and future therapeutic approaches. Biomed Eng Online 2021;20:24.
12. Lindsey BA, Markel JE, Kleinerman ES. Osteosarcoma Overview. Rheumatol Ther 2017;4(1):25–43.
13. Patel SR. Soft tissue and bone sarcoma and bone metastasis. In: Loscolzo J, Fauci A, Kasper D, et al, editors. Harrison's Principal of Internal medicine. 21st edition. McGraw Hill; 2022. Available at: https://accessmedicine.mhmedical.com/content.aspx?bookid=3095&sectionid=263547302. Accessed October 20, 2022.
14. Savage SA, Mirabello L. Using epidemiology and genomics to understand osteosarcoma etiology. Sarcoma 2011;2011:548151.
15. Menendez N, Epelman M, Shao L, et al. Pediatric Osteosarcoma: Pearls and Pitfalls. Semin Ultrasound CT MR 2022;43(1):97–114.
16. Mutsaers AJ, Walkley CJ. Cells of origin in osteosarcoma: Mesenchymal stem cells or osteoblast committed cells? Bone 2014;62:56–63.
17. Ferguson JL, Turner SP. Bone Cancer: Diagnosis and Treatment Principles. Am Fam Physician 2018;98(4):205–13.
18. Rothzerg E, Pfaff AL, Koks S. Innovative approaches for treatment of osteosarcoma. Exp Biol Med 2022;247(4):310–6.
19. Reed DR, Hayashi M, Wagner L, et al. Treatment pathway of bone sarcoma in children, adolescents, and young adults. Cancer 2017;123(12):2206–18.
20. Desai SS, Jambhekar NA. Pathology of Ewing's sarcoma/PNET: Current opinion and emerging concepts. Indian J Orthop 2010;44(4):363–8.
21. DuBois SG, Krailo MD, Gebhardt MC, et al. Comparative evaluation of local control strategies in localized Ewing sarcoma of bone: A report from the Children's Oncology Group. Cancer 2015;121:467–75.
22. Kim JH, Lee SK. Classification of Chondrosarcoma: From Characteristic to Challenging Imaging Findings. Cancers 2023;15:1703.
23. Tiemsani C, Larousserie F, De Percin S, et al. Biology and Management of High-Grade Chondrosarcoma: An Update on Targets and Treatment Options. Int J Mol Sci 2023;24:1361.
24. Italiano A, Mir O, Cioffi A, et al. Advanced chondrosarcomas: role of chemotherapy and survival. Ann Oncol 2013;24(11):2916–22.
25. Abbas K, Siddiqui AT. Evaluation of different treatment and management options for chondrosarcoma; the prognostic factors determining the outcome of the disease. Int J Surg: Oncology 2018;3(3):e85.
26. RIggi N, Suva ML, Stamenkovic I. Ewing's Sarcoma. N Engl J Med 2021;384:154–64. https://doi.org/10.1056/NEJMra2028910.
27. Kubo T, Furuta T, Johan MP, et al. A meta-analysis supports core needle biopsy by radiologists for better histological diagnosis in soft tissue and bone sarcomas. Medicine 2018;97(29):e11567.
28. Jawad MU, Scully SP. In brief: classifications in brief: Enneking classification: benign and malignant tumors of the musculoskeletal system. Clin Orthop Relat Res 2010;468(7):2000–2.
29. Rickel K, Fang F, Tao J. Molecular genetics of osteosarcoma. Bone 2017;102:69–79.
30. Jafari F, Javdansirat S, Sanaie S, et al. Osteosarcoma: A comprehensive review of management and treatment strategies. Ann Diagn Pathol 2020;49:1092–9134.
31. Ilaslon H, Schils J, Nageatee W, et al. Clinical presentation and imaging in bone and soft tissue sarcomas. Clev Clin J Med 2010;77(Suppl 1):S2–7.

32. Doyle LA. Sarcoma classification: An update based on 2013 World Health Organization Classification of Tumors of Soft Tissue and Bone. Cancer 2014;120(12): 1763–74.
33. Durfee RA, Mohammed M, Luu HH. Review of Osteosarcoma and Current Management. Rheumatol Ther 2016;3(2):221–43.
34. Meltzer PS, Helman LJ. New Horizons in the Treatment of Osteosarcoma. N Engl J Med 2021;385(22):2066–76.
35. Harris MA, Hawkins CJ. Recent and Ongoing Research into Metastatic Osteosarcoma Treatments. Int J Mol Sci 2022;23(7):3817.
36. Bosma SE, Ayu O, Fiocco M, et al. Prognostic factors for survival in Ewing sarcoma: A systematic review. Surgical Oncology 2018;27(4):603–10.
37. Gargallo P, Yáñez Y, Juan A, et al. Review: Ewing Sarcoma Predisposition. Pathol Oncol Res 2020;26:2057–66.
38. Mackintosh C, Madoz-Gúrpide J, Ordóñez JL, et al. The molecular pathogenesis of Ewing sarcoma. Cancer Biol Ther 2010;9:655–67.
39. Van Mater D, Wagner L. Management of recurrent Ewing's sarcoma: challenges and approaches. OncoTargets Ther 2019;12:2279–88.
40. Aran V, Devalle S, Meohas W, et al. Osteosarcoma, chondrosarcoma, and Ewing sarcoma: Clinical aspects, biomarker discovery, and liquid biopsy. Crit Rev Oncol Hematol 2021;162. https://doi.org/10.1016/j.critrevonc.2021.103340.
41. Nguyen MT, Jiang YQ, Li XL, et al. Risk Factors for Incidence and Prognosis in Chondrosarcoma Patients with Pulmonary Metastasis at Initial Diagnosis. Med Sci Monit 2019;25:10136–53.
42. Chow WA. Chondrosarcoma: biology, genetics, and epigenetics [version 1; peer review: 2 approved]. F1000Research 2018;7:1826.
43. Mendenhall WM, Reith JD, Scarborough MT, et al. Mesenchymal Chondrosarcoma. Int J Part Ther 2016l;3(2):300–4.
44. Mery B, Espenel E, Guy JB, et al. Biological aspects of chondrosarcoma: Leaps and hurdles. Crit Rev Oncol Hematol 2018;126:32–6.
45. Van Praag V, Rueten-Budde AJ, Ho V, et al. Incidence, outcomes, and prognostic factors during 25 years of treatment of chondrosarcoma. Surgical Oncology 2018;27(3):402–8.

Numbness and Tingling, Where Is It Coming From?

A Peripheral Neuropathy Overview for the New Orthopedic, Neurology, and Rehabilitation Clinician

Amy Dix, PhD, PA-C[a,b],*, Stephanie Kubiak, PhD, OTR/L[b]

KEYWORDS

- Orthopedic surgery–related neuropathy • Mononeuropathies • Polyneuropathies
- Neurology • Occupational therapy • Peripheral neuropathy • Neuropathic pain

KEY POINTS

- Iatrogenic and noniatrogenic mononeuropathies, mononeuropathy multiplex, and polyneuropathies can be seen in orthopedic clinical practice.
- Development of postsurgical neuropathy can be complicated by underlying common comorbidities (eg, diabetes and low B12).
- Pharmacologic treatment options for neuropathic symptoms are limited.
- Occupational therapy is a rehabilitative profession that can treat motor, sensory, and functional deficits experienced by a person living with neuropathy.

INTRODUCTION

Damage to one or more peripheral nerve fibers is defined as peripheral neuropathy.[1] Neuropathy can be found across specialties including primary care, neurology, pain management, and orthopedics. In this article, the authors provide a basic overview of nerve anatomy and function, the different presentations and causes of neuropathy, common neuropathies seen in orthopedic surgery settings, diagnostic procedures, and conservative treatment approaches. Then, using 2 upper extremity orthopedic case studies, diagnostic and treatment techniques are applied.

WHAT IS A NERVE AND HOW DOES IT WORK?
Nerve Anatomy and Function Overview

Nerves are similar to electrical cables that provide a signal between the brain and the rest of the body.[2] A human nerve cell (neuron) consists of an axon (sends signals), cell

[a] Cara Therapeutics; [b] Department of Occupational Therapy, Gannon University, 109 University Square Erie, PA 16541, USA
* Corresponding author.
E-mail address: Ald7273@gmail.com

Physician Assist Clin 9 (2024) 109–121
https://doi.org/10.1016/j.cpha.2023.07.011
2405-7991/24/© 2023 Elsevier Inc. All rights reserved.

physicianassistant.theclinics.com

body (controls cellular functions), and dendrites (receives signals). Axons (myelinated or unmyelinated) are what makes up a nerve fiber, which can vary in size and are responsible for sending electrical impulses (eg, sensory or motor signals) away from the cell body to other neurons.[1] Speed of the electrical impulse is determined by the presence or absence of a protective axonal myelin sheath (Schwann cells). A myelinated nerve transmits electrical signals faster.[1] Myelinated and unmyelinated nerves are further differentiated by their function, consisting of motor, sensory, or autonomic types. In the next section the authors review the 3 types of nerve fibers.

Nerve Fibers

Nerve branches are made up of motor, *sensory*, or autonomic nerve fibers.[1] Motor nerve fibers are responsible for transmitting efferent signals from the central nervous system to specific muscle groups. Muscle weakness is a symptom of motor neuropathy. Typically, signs of a motor neuropathy can include problems with coordination, walking, swallowing, and talking.[1]

Sensory nerve fibers transmit afferent sensory signals (eg, pain, temperature, balance, touch, and so forth) from parts of the body back to the central nervous system (brain and spinal cord). Large sensory fibers are responsible for sending joint position (proprioception), balance, and touch signals.[3] Small sensory fibers are responsible for sending itch and pain signals.[3] Symptoms present as distortion of cutaneous touch (dysesthesias) and can include distal numbness, tingling, itching, or pain from nerve impingement, trauma, or irritation.[1] The physical examination may show diminution or loss of sensation to pin prick, temperature, or vibratory perception as well as loss of proprioception in hands or feet.

Autonomic nerve fibers are responsible for innervating or sending signals to and from organs within the body, contributing to heart rate, bowel and bladder, and other bodily functions.[1] Examples of autonomic dysfunction include orthostasis (including orthostatic hypotension) and gastroparesis.[4] A summary of neuropathy symptoms by nerve fiber type is described in **Fig. 1**.

CLASSIFICATION OF PERIPHERAL NEUROPATHY DISORDERS

Peripheral neuropathies include a wide range of disorders that can affect one or many nerves with deficits presenting in unique patterns.[5] The pattern of neuropathy deficits can be classified as either mononeuropathy (focal nerve damage), mononeuropathy

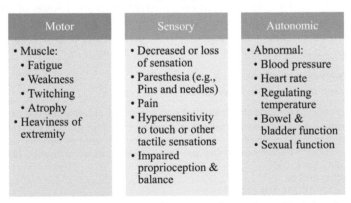

Motor	Sensory	Autonomic

• Muscle:
  • Fatigue
  • Weakness
  • Twitching
  • Atrophy
• Heaviness of extremity
	• Decreased or loss of sensation
	• Paresthesia (e.g., Pins and needles)
	• Pain
	• Hypersensitivity to touch or other tactile sensations
	• Impaired proprioception & balance
		• Abnormal:
		  • Blood pressure
		  • Heart rate
		  • Regulating temperature
		  • Bowel & bladder function
		  • Sexual function

Fig. 1. Neuropathy symptoms by nerve fiber type. (*Data from* "Peripheral neuropathy: When the numbness, weakness and pain won't stop" by N. Latov, Demos Medical Publishing. Copyright (2007) by AAN Enterprises.[1])

multiplex (multifocal nerve damage), or polyneuropathy generalized nerve damage.[1] When one nerve is damaged, this is defined as mononeuropathy or focal neuropathy (eg, a single nerve entrapment injury). Multifocal injuries, also called mononeuropathy multiplex, involve more than one peripheral nerve that can affect bilateral extremities but can be asymmetrical in their presentation (eg, vasculitis). Generalized neuropathy or polyneuropathy involves more than one peripheral nerve and follows a symmetric pattern (eg, Guillain-Barré syndrome).[6] Now the authors elaborate on each of the peripheral neuropathy presentations. See **Fig. 2** for examples of common diagnoses by neuropathy type.

Focal Mononeuropathy

Mononeuropathy is a focal nerve injury with sensorimotor deficits isolated to the affected nerve's distribution and can occur in the upper or lower extremities.[1] It is typically a result of entrapment (compressed nerve), palsy (nerve inflammation), or injury of a single peripheral nerve.[1] Examples include carpal tunnel syndrome, ulnar neuropathy, pronator teres or anterior interosseous syndrome, femoral neuropathy, meralgia paresthetica, sciatic and fibular (common peroneal) nerve palsies, tarsal tunnel syndrome, and compressive neuropathy of the upper arm or axilla ("Saturday night palsy").[4]

Mononeuropathy Multiplex

Mononeuropathy multiplex or multifocal nerve injury is a result of vascular, immunologic, or infectious processes.[4] This type of neuropathy exhibits a combination of motor, sensory, and/or autonomic deficits that affect individual adjacent nerves versus a diffuse and/or symmetric nerve pattern (eg, polyneuropathy). Mononeuropathy multiplex cause includes vasculopathy (eg, arteritis), infiltration process (eg, leprosy, sarcoidosis), radiation damage, or immunologic disorders (eg, brachial plexopathy).[4]

Polyneuropathy

Polyneuropathy consists of sensory, motor, autonomic, or a combination (mixed) pattern of deficits typically occurring in the distal extremities.[1] Polyneuropathy often exhibits distal extremity weakness and sensation, absent or impaired tendon reflexes, pain, muscle tenderness, itching, numbness, and/or tingling (paresthesias).[4] Common types and causes of polyneuropathy include genetic neuropathies, metabolic, toxin, idiopathic inflammatory polyneuropathy (eg, Guillain- Barré syndrome), diabetes, and malignant disease.[1] Underlying polyneuropathy conditions (eg, diabetes) are a risk factor for postoperative complications (including orthopedic surgeries) and worse outcomes after surgery.[7,8]

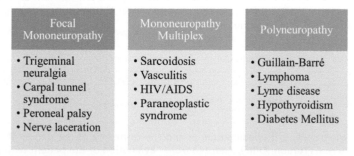

Focal Mononeuropathy	Mononeuropathy Multiplex	Polyneuropathy
• Trigeminal neuralgia • Carpal tunnel syndrome • Peroneal palsy • Nerve laceration	• Sarcoidosis • Vasculitis • HIV/AIDS • Paraneoplastic syndrome	• Guillain-Barré • Lymphoma • Lyme disease • Hypothyroidism • Diabetes Mellitus

Fig. 2. Examples of peripheral neuropathy types and diagnoses. (*Data from* "Peripheral neuropathies: A practical approach" by M. Bromberg, 2018, Cambridge University Press (doi.org/10.1017/9781316135815). Copyright (2018) by M. Bromberg.[4])

POSTSURGICAL NEUROPATHY

Orthopedic clinicians may see a new onset of neuropathy symptoms in the postsurgical setting or may discover an underlying neuropathy condition. Nerve damage occurring as a result of surgery is called an iatrogenic nerve injury.[9] Orthopedic surgeries are responsible for approximately 20% of traumatic peripheral nerve injuries,[10,11] with ulnar nerve and brachial plexus injuries being the most common.[9] Iatrogenic nerve injuries can be a result of direct injuries (eg, nerve lacerations from placing or removing joints, implants, or pins) or indirect injuries (eg, compression, thermal, traction, or stretch of a nerve). A review of common upper extremity orthopedic surgical procedures and the corresponding at-risk nerves can be found in **Figs. 3** and **4**.

Orthopedic providers should consult with the neurology team to diagnose and oversee neuropathy treatment. The process of diagnosing peripheral neuropathy consists of a physical examination, laboratory studies, imaging, and an electromyogram (including nerve conduction and muscle evaluation).[12] Sometimes, neuromuscular specialists or dermatologists may perform nerve or skin biopsies to determine cause of complex neuropathies. **Figs. 5** and **6** provide a summary of the elements of a neuropathy evaluation.

If an iatrogenic nerve injury after orthopedic surgery is suspected, first an in-depth clinical history and physical examination can assist with localizing the nerve lesion. Clinical history should investigate the patient's reported symptoms and timeline of events before and after their surgery.[11] A mononeuropathy evaluation is important, and a physical examination should include a thorough neurologic and musculoskeletal assessment of the affected extremity.

If an iatrogenic nerve injury is ruled out, other neuropathy causes should be explored. "Dang Therapist" is a useful acronym that can be used to outline common premorbid and nonsurgery-related causes of neuropathy (**Fig. 7**).[13] Most common causes of non-iatrogenic peripheral neuropathies include diabetes and B12 deficiency.[5,14]

MANAGEMENT

If nerve damage is present, balancing the expected spontaneous recovery (nerve regeneration of approximately one inch per month) with the need of surgical or conservative interventions must be considered.[11] If warranted, neuropathy treatment (conservative or surgical) should be initiated as soon as possible for best outcomes.[16]

Reversible Causes of Neuropathy

When neuropathy is suspected, reversible causes of surgery-associated nerve injuries need to be eliminated. Fixing a poor fitting device, such as a cast, splint, or dressing, should come first. Other reversible causes include implant entrapment or hematoma, and, in these cases, early intervention is recommended.[11] Intervention planning is critical and may require a neurology consult.

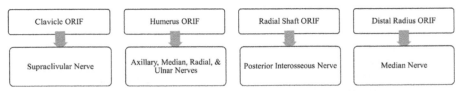

Fig. 3. Upper extremity orthopedic surgeries and the respective at-risk nerves. (*Note.* Open Reduction Internal Fixation (ORIF); *Adapted from* "Evaluation of the patient with postoperative peripheral nerve issues" by M. Shlykov, K. Velicki, and C. Dy, 2021, In C. Dy, D. Brogan, and E. Wagner (Eds.), *Peripheral Nerve Issues after Orthopedic Surgery: A Multidisciplinary Approach to Prevention, Evaluation and Treatment*, p. 28, Springer Publishing (https://link.springer.com/chapter/10.1007/978-3-030-84428-8_2). Copyright (2022) by Springer Nature.[11])

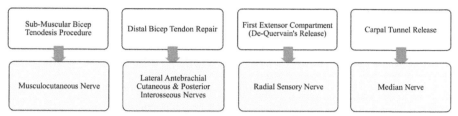

Fig. 4. Other upper extremity surgeries and the respective at-risk nerves. (*Adapted from* "Evaluation of the patient with postoperative peripheral nerve issues" by M. Shlykov, K. Velicki, and C. Dy, 2021, In C. Dy, D. Brogan, and E. Wagner (Eds.), *Peripheral Nerve Issues after Orthopedic Surgery: A Multidisciplinary Approach to Prevention, Evaluation and Treatment*, p. 28, Springer Publishing (https://link.springer.com/chapter/10.1007/978-3-030-84428-8_2). Copyright (2022) by Springer Nature.[11])

Nonsurgical Neuropathy Management

Pharmacologic management of neuropathy addresses neuropathic symptoms. Despite the prevalence of neuropathy, few treatment options exist. Oral therapies for neuropathy are often used off-label.[17] The following categories of agents are used in clinical practice and include tricyclic antidepressants such as amitriptyline and nortriptyline, antiepileptics such as gabapentin and pregabalin, selective serotonin reuptake inhibitors such as duloxetine and venlafaxine, and lidocaine patches.[5]

Only duloxetine and pregabalin have been approved by the Food and Drug Administration for the treatment of diabetic neuropathic pain. Yet prescribers often start with gabapentin, amitriptyline, or nortriptyline due to cost because they share a similar mechanism of action.[5] Opioids can be used to treat neuropathic pain; however, because they are a controlled substance with addictive side effects they are rarely used as a first-line treatment and are often saved for second- or third-line treatments.[5]

In addition to pharmacologic management, complementary and alternative therapies can also be used. Nearly 50% of people living with peripheral neuropathy use complementary and/or alternative medicine including acupuncture, vitamin supplementation, and herbal remedies. Use of implantable devices for pain management are also available.[5]

Treatment of the underlying autoimmune disease–causing neuropathy can improve symptom management.[5] Autoimmune neuropathies are treated with immunomodulating agents such as azathioprine, cyclophosphamide, cyclosporin, mycophenolate, and methotrexate. New-onset postsurgical neuropathy changes can be treated with corticosteroid to reduce local inflammation. Corticosteroids can also be used to treat vascular or immunogenic neuropathy. Finally, for the treatment of acute neurogenic neuropathic symptoms (eg, chronic inflammatory demyelinating polyneuropathy) plasmaphereses is used if patients are unresponsive to corticosteroids.[5]

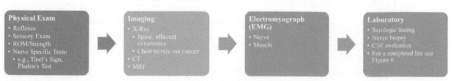

Fig. 5. Neuropathy evaluation. (*Data from* "Peripheral neuropathy: Evaluation and differential diagnosis" by G. Castelli, K. Desai, and R. Cantone, 2020, *American Academy of Family Physicians*, *102*(12), 732-739 (https://www.aafp.org/pubs/afp/issues/2020/1215/p732.html). Copyright (2020) American Academy of Family Physicians.[12])

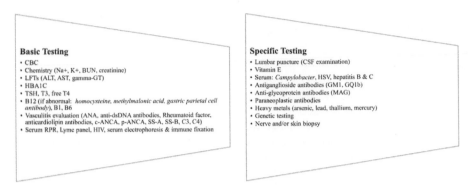

Basic Testing
- CBC
- Chemistry (Na+, K+, BUN, creatinine)
- LFTs (ALT, AST, gamma-GT)
- HBA1C
- TSH, T3, free T4
- B12 (if abnormal: *homocysteine, methylmalonic acid, gastric parietal cell antibody*), B1, B6
- Vasculitis evaluation (ANA, anti-dsDNA antibodies, Rheumatoid factor, anticardiolipin antibodies, c-ANCA, p-ANCA, SS-A, SS-B, C3, C4)
- Serum RPR, Lyme panel, HIV, serum electrophoresis & immune fixation

Specific Testing
- Lumbar puncture (CSF examination)
- Vitamin E
- Serum: *Campylobacter*, HSV, hepatitis B & C
- Antiganglioside antibodies (GM1, GQ1b)
- Anti-glycoprotein antibodies (MAG)
- Paraneoplastic antibodies
- Heavy metals (arsenic, lead, thallium, mercury)
- Genetic testing
- Nerve and/or skin biopsy

Fig. 6. Diagnostic and laboratory evaluation of neuropathy. ANA, antinuclear antibody test; anti-dsDNA antibodies, anti–double-stranded DNA used to help diagnosis lupus; anti-SSA and -SSB, antinuclear antibodies, B12, vitamin B12; C3, complement 3 protein; C4, compliment 4 protein; c-ANCA, antineutrophil cytoplasmic antibodies; CBC, complete blood count; CSF, cerebral spinal fluid; GM1, monosialotetrahexosylganglioside important in neuronal plasticity and repair; GQ1b, antiganglioside antibody; HbA1C, hemoglobin A1C; HIV, human immunodeficiency virus; HSV, herpes simplex virus; LFT, liver function test; MAG, myelin-associated glycoprotein; P-ANCA, perinuclear antineutrophil cytoplasmic antibodies; RPR, rapid plasma reagin screening test for syphilis; T3, triiodothyronine test; T4, thyroxine; TSH, thyroid-stimulating hormone. (*Adapted from Fundamentals of neurology: An illustrated guide* (2nd ed.) by H. Mattle and M. Mumenthaler, 2016, p. 280, Thieme Publishing (https://shop.thieme.com/Fundamentals-of-Neurology/9783131364524). Copyright (2016) Thieme Publishing.[15])

D	Diabetic
A	Alcohol
N	Nutritional (vitamins, B6, B12)
G	Guillain-Barre Syndrome
T	Toxic (lead, arsenic, vinblastine other)
He	Hereditary
R	Recurrent
A	Amyloid
P	Porphyria (motor , involvement, intermittent)
I	Infections (AIDS, mononucleosis, leprosy, diphtheria)
S	Systemic (CVD, uremia dysproteinemias)
T	Tumor (paraneoplastic)

Fig. 7. Acronym for common causes of noniatrogenic neuropathy. (*Adapted from* "Neuromuscular Disorders. In D. Gelb (Ed.), *Introduction to Clinical Neurology* (5th ed.)" by M. Bromberg and D. Gelb, 2016, pp. 200-201, Oxford University Press. Copyright (2016) by Oxford University Press.[13])

REHABILITATION

Functional and physical deficits and the rehabilitation approaches vary depending on number of nerves affected, types of nerve or nerves affected (sensory, motor, and/or autonomic), and extremities involved. Upper extremity peripheral neuropathy can cause difficulties with daily self-care and work-related tasks due to pain, weakness, and/or sensory deficits.[18] To address these functional deficits, an occupational therapy consultation is recommended.

Occupational therapy is a profession that provides rehabilitation treatment across the lifespan with the primary goal of promoting participation and independence in "everyday life occupations" [(p. 1)].[19] Occupations can include daily self-care tasks (eg, dressing, bathing, cooking, cleaning, and so forth), sleep, education, work, play, leisure, and social participation.[19] When evaluating a new client, occupational therapy practitioners (OTP) will ask a client to describe their reported symptoms, difficulties in occupations, current roles, routines, environment, and goals. Next, the OTP will analyze a client's occupational performance abilities, including motor, sensory, cognitive, and social abilities, and deficits. Based on all these factors, an intervention plan would be developed that could include rehabilitation, compensatory, environmental adaptations, prevention, preservation of function, and/or health promotion or well-being intervention approaches.[19]

After an upper extremity nerve impairment or neuropathy, it is recommended to initiate treatment (conservative or surgical) as soon as possible, as prolonged time to initiate treatment predicts greater disability and worse functional outcomes.[16] Common deficits of upper extremity peripheral nerve impairments include sleep difficulties, weakness, sensory impairments, negative changes to mental health, difficulty completing work and home tasks, pain, and negative impacts on social and intimate relationships.[18] All these functional deficits are within the occupational therapy scope of practice.[19] Referral to occupational therapy can be an efficient and effective approach to treating the physical, functional, and mental health deficits reported by clients with upper extremity peripheral neuropathy. Next, the authors apply neuropathy evaluation procedures and conservative treatment approaches to 2 orthopedic case studies.

CASE STUDY EXAMPLE 1: MONONEUROPATHY
Background

A 43-year-old right-handed, senior executive presents to an outpatient orthopedic clinic. The patient reports new-onset right hand paresthesias in digits 4 and 5. The patient had previously been working in an office setting before COVID 19 global pandemic, when she transitioned to working remotely. Other symptoms reported include right trapezius pain, new-onset hand weakness, difficulty opening jars, dropping objects while cooking, and pain in her hand and digits. Dynamometry testing indicates the patient's right grip strength is less than normal. The patient describes her work set-up as a small desk, laptop without use of a mouse, and nonadjustable kitchen chair without back support while working 10+ hours a day at her workstation with minimal breaks. **Table 1** provides a summary of the evaluation and treatment of Case Study 1. After the initial patient visit the orthopedic provider consulted neurology and the following case consists of a collaboration between neurology and orthopedic services. The patient was found to have mild cervical degenerative disk disease along with both radial and ulnar neuropathy and B12 deficiency. A conservative therapeutic approach was initiated, which included an occupational therapy consult, Lidoderm patch, and splinting.

Table 1
Case study 1: evaluation and treatment

Evaluation Process

Symptoms	Differential diagnosis[20]	Examination, Diagnostics, & Relevant findings[12]	Diagnosis

Right sided:
• Paresthesia digits 4 & 5
• Upper trapezius pain
• Hand weakness
• Pain in hand and digits
• Dropping items, possibly sensory deficits
	• Cervical radiculopathy
	• Carpal tunnel
	• Ulnar neuropathy
	• Demyelinating disorders
		• Physical examination
		• Right hand strength
		  ○ Below norms
		• Right hand sensation
		  ○ Diminished pin prick
		• Right Tinel & Phalen tests
		  ○ Positive
		• EMG of right upper extremity (Neurology referral)
		  ○ Slower electrical responses at cubital tunnel indicating compression of ulnar nerve
		  ○ Slowing of the median nerve velocity across the wrist
		• Laboratory testing
		  ○ CBC, chemistry, folate, hepatitis panel, ESR, ANA, & TSH all WNL
		  ○ Low B12 (<250 ng/ml)
		• MRI
		  ○ Slight cervical degenerative changes at C4-C5
			• Right ulnar entrapment at elbow (ulnar neuropathy)
			• Right mild carpal tunnel at wrist (median neuropathy)
			• Slight cervical degenerative changes at C4-C5
			• B12 deficiency

Treatment Plan

Medical Treatment:	OT Evaluation[19]:	OT Treatment Overview:

• Wrist splint at night[21]
• Lidoderm patch under splint at nighttime[22]
• Referral to occupational therapy evaluation and treatment[19]
  ○ Ergonomic evaluation
  ○ Wrist splint fabrication and fitting
    ○ ADL & IADLs
• B12[23]
	• Ergonomic workstation evaluation
	• Assess upper extremity range of motion, strength, sensation, and coordination
	• ADLs and IADLs including cooking and work-related tasks
		• Workstation recommendations[24]:
		  ○ Adjust keyboard and mouse locations
		  ○ Elevating dual monitors to be eye level
		  ○ Office chair seat at a height where at least 90° hip and knee flexion can be obtained while feet are flat on the floor
		  ○ Lumbar support
		• Wrist splint fabrication, fitting, and training of nocturnal wear schedule[21]
		• Exercise to improve ROM, strength, pain, numbness, and tingling in digits and hand[21]
		  ○ Tendon and nerve glides
		  ○ Kinesio taping
		  ○ ROM and digit-strengthening exercises
		• Adapted equipment education (eg, adapted jar opener, built up handles) to ease independence with ADLs[25]

Abbreviations: ADL, activities of daily living; CBC, complete blood count; EMG, electromyography; ESR, erythrocyte sedimentation rate; IADL, instrumental activities of daily living; MRI, magnetic resonance imaging; OT, occupational therapy; ROM, and range of motion; TSH, thyroid-stimulating hormone; WNL, within normal limits.

Table 2
Case study 2: evaluation and treatment

Evaluation Process

Symptoms	Differential Diagnosis[20]	Examination, Diagnostics, & Relevant Findings[12]	Diagnoses

Bilateral upper extremity
• Hand weakness
• Pruritis
• Palmar numbness
• Tingling in hands
Left upper extremity residual swelling from postoperative infection
	Peripheral cause
	• Nerve entrapment at surgical site
	• Postsurgical nerve changes
	• Bilateral carpal tunnel
	• Ulnar neuropathy
	• Radial nerve palsy
	• Diabetic neuropathy
		Physical examination
		• Bilateral hand strength
		  ○ Below norms
		• Bilateral hand sensation
		  ○ Diminished pin prick
		• Tinel & Phalen tests
		  ○ Negative
		EMG (upper and lower extremities)
		• Bilateral peripheral neuropathy
		• Left radial mononeuropathy
		Laboratory test results (fasting)
		• Blood sugar of 126
		• HbA1c of 6.6%
			• Diabetes
			• Diabetic neuropathy
			• Left radial nerve palsy

Treatment Plan

Medical Treatment	OT Evaluation[19]	OT Treatment Overview[19]

• Collaborated with orthopedic and plan for conservative treatment approach of radial nerve palsy[26]
• Referral to primary care for diabetes management
• 300 mg gabapentin BID titrate to 600 mg for numbness and tingling[27]
• Referral to occupational therapy for evaluation and treatment:
  ○ Left UE ROM and strength
  ○ ADL
  ○ Diabetes management
	• Assess bilateral upper extremity range of motion, strength, sensation, and coordination
	• ADLs & IADLs and return-to-work evaluation[28]
	• Self-management of diabetes[29]
		• Radial nerve palsy rehabilitation
		  ○ Ultrasound, electrical stimulation, heat, manual therapy, upper extremity range-of-motion and strength exercises (while maintaining any orthopedic postsurgical precautions)[30]
		• Education and training on the self-management of diabetes[29,31]
		  ○ Goal setting; education of diabetes disease management and progression; health promotion, navigating the health care system; identifying social support systems (eg, diabetic community); stress management and coping skills; long-term planning[29]
		• Bilateral hand and foot diabetic home exercise program[31]
		• Target performance to improve independence with ADLs, IADLs, and tasks required to return to floor laying
		  ○ Joint mobility, muscle power, muscle endurance, and muscle control and coordination[28]

Abbreviations: ADL, activities of daily living; BID, twice a day; EMG, electromyography; HbA1c, hemoglobin A1C; IADL, instrumental activities of daily living; OT, occupational therapy; ROM, range of motion; UE, upper extremity.

CASE STUDY EXAMPLE 2: POLYNEUROPATHY
Background

A 55-year-old, left hand dominate experienced a fall off a ladder while cleaning leaves out of his gutters. He sustained a left closed distal humeral fracture and underwent an open reduction internal fixation (ORIF) procedure 2 months ago. He presents to ortho for a follow-up with a concern of decreased bilateral hand strength, pruritis, numbness, and tingling. Dynamometry testing shows bilateral grip strength below normal limits (10 pounds on left and 12 pounds on the right). The sensory examination revealed diminished pin prick on bilateral palmar surfaces of hands. Incision from ORIF became infected 2 weeks postsurgery and required antibiotics. **Table 2** provides a summary of the evaluation and treatment of Case Study 2. The patient was found to have left radial nerve palsy and diabetic neuropathy. A conservative therapeutic approach was initiated, which included an occupational therapy consult, pharmacologic management, and primary care referral for diabetes management.

SUMMARY

Diagnosis and treatment of mono- and polyneuropathy is an important aspect of orthopedic management. Orthopedic providers should be aware of iatrogenic nerve injury risk during surgery, in addition to other underlying neuropathies (eg, diabetes) that may complicate postsurgical outcomes. Interdisciplinary care between orthopedic and neurology providers play an important role in diagnosing and treating neuropathy conditions, whereas occupational therapists can address functional impairments.

CLINICS CARE POINTS

- Peripheral nerves consist of motor, sensory, or autonomic nerve fibers.
- Peripheral neuropathy is a neurologic disorder affecting the peripheral nerves. Neuropathies can affect one or many nerves and are categorized as mononeuropathy, polyneuropathy, or mononeuropathy multiplex.
- "Dang-Therapist" is an acronym for common noniatrogenic causes of neuropathy.
- If nerve damage is present, balancing the expected spontaneous recovery (nerve regeneration of approximately 1 inch per month) with the need of surgical or conservative interventions must be considered.
- Care coordination between orthopedic, neurology, and occupational therapy is an opportunity for best practice.

CONFLICT OF INTEREST

The authors have no conflicts of interest to disclose.

REFERENCES

1. Latov N. Peripheral neuropathy: "When the numbness, weakness and pain won't stop". NYC, New York: Demos Medical Publishing; 2007.
2. Muzio M, Cascella M. Histology, axon. StatPearls Publishing; 2023. Available at: https://www.ncbi.nlm.nih.gov/books/NBK554388/.
3. Oaklander AL. Neuropathic Itch. Semin Cutan Med Surg 2011;30(2):87–92.
4. Bromberg M. Peripheral neuropathies: a practical approach. Cambridge, England: Cambridge University Press; 2018.

5. Barrell K, Smith AG. Peripheral Neuropathy. Med Clin North Am 2019;103(2): 383–97.
6. Poncelet AN. An algorithm for the evaluation of peripheral neuropathy. Am Fam Physician 1998;57(4):755–64.
7. Kennedy JM, Zochodne DW. Impaired peripheral nerve regeneration in diabetes mellitus. J Peripher Nerv Syst 2005;10(2):144–57.
8. Martin ET, Kaye KS, Knott C, et al. Diabetes and Risk of Surgical Site Infection: A Systematic Review and Meta-analysis. Infect Control Hosp Epidemiol 2016;37(1): 88–99.
9. Zhang J, Moore AE, Stringer MD. Iatrogenic upper limb nerve injuries: a systematic review. ANZ J Surg 2011;81(4):227–36.
10. Kretschmer T, Antoniadis G, Braun V, et al. Evaluation of iatrogenic lesions in 722 surgically treated cases of peripheral nerve trauma. J Neurosurg 2001;94(6): 905–12.
11. Shlykov M, Velicki K, Dy C. Evaluation of the patient with postoperative peripheral nerve issues. In: Dy CJ, Brogan DM, Wagner ER, editors. Peripheral nerve issues after orthopedic surgery: a multidisciplinary approach to prevention, evaluation and treatment. New York: Springer International Publishing; NYC; 2021. p. 27–40.
12. Castelli G, Desai KM, Cantone RE. Peripheral Neuropathy: Evaluation and Differential Diagnosis. Am Fam Physician 2020;102(12):732–9.
13. Bromberg M, Gelb D. Neuromuscular disorders. In: Gelb D, editor. *Introduction to clinical neurology.* 5th edition. Oxford, England: Oxford University Press; 2016. p. 185–210.
14. Leishear K, Boudreau RM, Studenski SA, et al. Relationship Between Vitamin B12 and Sensory and Motor Peripheral Nerve Function in Older Adults. J Am Geriatr Soc 2012;60(6):1057–63.
15. Mattle H, Mumenthaler M. Fundamentals of Neurology: An Illustrated Guide. Thieme 2016.
16. Stonner MM, Mackinnon SE, Kaskutas V. Predictors of functional outcome after peripheral nerve injury and compression. J Hand Ther 2021;34(3):369–75.
17. Azhary H, Farooq MU, Bhanushali M, et al. Peripheral neuropathy: differential diagnosis and management. Am Fam Physician 2010;81(7):887–92.
18. Stonner MM, Mackinnon SE, Kaskutas V. Predictors of Disability and Quality of Life With an Upper-Extremity Peripheral Nerve Disorder. Am J Occup Ther 2017;71(1):1–8.
19. American Occupational Therapy Association. Occupational therapy practice framework: Domain and process. Am J Occup Ther 2020;74(Supplement 2). https://doi.org/10.5014/ajot.2020.74s2001.
20. Smith SM, McMullen CW, Herring SA. Differential Diagnosis for the Painful Tingling Arm. Curr Sports Med Rep 2021;20(9):462–9.
21. Nazarieh M, Hakakzadeh A, Ghannadi S, et al. Non-Surgical Management and Post-Surgical Rehabilitation of Carpal Tunnel Syndrome: An Algorithmic Approach and Practical Guideline. Asian J Sports Med 2020;11(3):1–13.
22. Nalamachu S, Crockett RS, Mathur D. Lidocaine patch 5 for carpal tunnel syndrome: how it compares with injections: a pilot study. J Fam Pract 2006;55(3): 209–14.
23. Baute V, Zelnik D, Curtis J, et al. Complementary and Alternative Medicine for Painful Peripheral Neuropathy. Curr Treat Options Neurol 2019;21(9). https://doi.org/10.1007/s11940-019-0584-z.

24. Woo EHC, White P, Lai CWK. Ergonomics standards and guidelines for computer workstation design and the impact on users' health – a review. Ergonomics 2016; 59(3):464–75.

25. Rahman K, Haque E, Bhuiyan T, et al. A study of forty patients of carpal tunnel syndrome. Journal of Dental and Medical Sciences 2018;17(3):25–34.

26. Hendrickx LAM, Hilgersom NFJ, Alkaduhimi H, et al. Radial nerve palsy associated with closed humeral shaft fractures: a systematic review of 1758 patients. Arch Orthop Trauma Surg 2021;141(4):561–8.

27. Newman P. Diabetes-related sensory peripheral neuropathy. Diabetes Prim Care 2022;24(6):187–90.

28. Blas AJT, Beltran KMB, Martinez PGV, et al. Enabling Work: Occupational Therapy Interventions for Persons with Occupational Injuries and Diseases: A Scoping Review. J Occup Rehabil 2018;28(2):201–14.

29. Pyatak EA, Carandang K, Vigen CLP, et al. Occupational Therapy Intervention Improves Glycemic Control and Quality of Life Among Young Adults With Diabetes: the Resilient, Empowered, Active Living with Diabetes (REAL Diabetes) Randomized Controlled Trial. Diabetes Care 2018;41(4):696–704.

30. Milicin C, Sîrbu E. A comparative study of rehabilitation therapy in traumatic upper limb peripheral nerve injuries. NeuroRehabilitation 2018;42(1):113–9.

31. Win MMTM, Fukai K, Nyunt HH, et al. Hand and foot exercises for diabetic peripheral neuropathy: A randomized controlled trial. Nurs Health Sci 2020;22(2):416–26.

Topics in Pediatric Orthopedics

Amy L. Noyes, MSN, CPNP, APRN RNFA,
Victoria Gentile, PA-C, MMSc, MA*, Katherine Holmes, MSN, APRN*

KEYWORDS

- Physis • Ossification • Scoliosis • Developmental dysplasia of the hip
- Slipped capital femoral epiphysis • Legg-calve-perthes • Genu valgum/varum
- Pediatric orthopedics

KEY POINTS

- Pediatric orthopedics presents unique challenges related to growth and development.
- Treating orthopedic conditions in the skeletally immature population requires familiarity with growth plates, primary and secondary ossification, and age-dependent bone characteristics.
- Pediatric-specific diagnoses such as physeal injuries, scoliosis, hip dysplasia, and limb deformity require specialized knowledge to avoid complications and mistreatment.
- This article will focus on how to identify and diagnose pediatric orthopedic issues and provide guidance on when to refer.

INTRODUCTION

Pediatric Orthopedics is a dynamic subspecialty encompassing musculoskeletal care of patients beginning with fetal development and continuing to skeletal maturity. At the core of pediatric orthopedics is an understanding of typical growth and development. From their joints and muscles to their motor and developmental capabilities, children are in a constant state of change. One must be able to adapt the assessment, diagnostic differential, and management for the patient's age and stage of development. This article outlines a few fundamental concepts and essential diagnoses in pediatric orthopedics.

Chapter Limitations

Unfortunately, an article of this length cannot cover all pediatric orthopedic topics. A particularly important omission of this review is non-accidental trauma (NAT). For any pediatric provider, it is essential to be familiar with findings concerning for child abuse

Yale New Haven Health Pediatric Orthopedics, 1 Long Wharf Drive, New Haven, CT 06511, USA
* Corresponding authors.
E-mail addresses: victoria.gentile@ynhh.org (V.G.); katherine.holmes@yale.edu (K.H.)

Physician Assist Clin 9 (2024) 123–135
https://doi.org/10.1016/j.cpha.2023.07.012
2405-7991/24/© 2023 Elsevier Inc. All rights reserved.

physicianassistant.theclinics.com

and neglect such as bruising in various stages of healing (especially on the head or torso), discordance between history and clinical findings, delay in seeking care, injury out of proportion to reported mechanism, fractures in non-ambulatory children, and specific fracture patterns that are highly suspicious for NAT (ex. metaphyseal corner fractures).[1] *PEARL: Any fracture in a non-ambulatory child and/or child less than 1 year of age should raise suspicion for NAT and prompt additional inquiry to rule out abuse.* This article does not include a detailed review of NAT but we implore readers to educate themselves on how to identify NAT if caring for young or vulnerable patient populations. The points referenced above provides a good initial overview. In addition, all pediatric providers are mandated reporters of suspected abuse and neglect, being familiar with state laws is also essential.

Ossification

Before discussing specific diagnoses, it will be beneficial to review some fundamental concepts. In growing bodies, there are primary and secondary endochondral ossification centers. Primary ossification centers eventually develop into the diaphyses of long bones while secondary ossification centers become the epiphyses of long bones. Secondary centers are of particular importance because their first appearances on x-ray (when they transition from radiolucent cartilage to radiopaque bone) occur throughout skeletal maturation. A great example is the pediatric elbow which has *six* different secondary ossification centers. As a patient matures, each of these centers ossifies separately and appears on x-ray at a different age.[2] These nascent bones can initially look fragmented and irregular on x-ray. Over time, they become dense and clearly corticated. A clinician unfamiliar with secondary ossification can easily misinterpret these centers as fractures or other pathologic osseous findings. *PEARL: One can distinguish a pathologic finding from a developmental variant by cross checking the patient's x-ray with a known normal x-ray of a child the same age, (there are online databases where one can easily access such x-rays),[3] by corroborating imaging with history and exam, or by imaging the contralateral extremity for comparison.*

Remodeling

Pediatric bones are unique in their ability to correct deformities over time. Osteoblasts and osteoclasts work sequentially to build and resorb bone. This process can reshape bones in response to injury. If there is malalignment at a fracture, there will be accelerated growth along the fracture concavity and resorption along the convexity, restoring the original shape of the bone.[4] The younger the patient, the more robust this process can be. An infant may heal and remodel a clavicle fracture in just a few weeks while the same fracture in a teenager may require months and never completely reshape. Pediatric orthopedists estimate how much remodeling potential a patient has based on various factors (age, appearance of growth plates, pubertal markers, proximity of the fracture site to the physis, and so forth) to devise an appropriate treatment plan. For example, an orthopedist may allow a transverse distal radius fracture with 15° of angulation in a 7-year-old to heal with this deformity because of the patient's high remodeling potential. The same fracture in a 15-year-old will require reduction and possibly surgery since there is not enough growth remaining to remodel the fracture. Unfortunately, no quick trick or algorithm exists to make these treatment decisions; understanding the nuances comes with experience.

Physeal Considerations

Physes, or growth plates, exist between the primary and secondary ossification centers. Physes are composed of cartilage and are responsible for longitudinal bone growth. They are present throughout the body in infancy and fuse at varying ages as an individual nears skeletal maturity (around age 16 in young women and 18 in young men). There are both acute and chronic diagnoses associated with physes. Salter-Harris fractures are fractures involving growth plates and are characterized by type depending on the position of the fracture relative to the growth plate. Some physeal injuries (fracture, infection, tumor, and so forth) require special attention because damage to the growth plate can result in altered growth at that site (**Fig. 1**).[5]

Case #1

An 11-year-old presents with acute knee pain, swelling, and inability to bear weight on the right leg. This began 45 minutes ago when he collided with another player during hockey practice. X-rays reveal a displaced Salter-Harris Type 2 fracture of the proximal tibia. The ER team reduces the fracture and applies a long leg cast. Follow up x-rays show anatomic fracture alignment. Over the next 12 weeks, the fracture heals and the patient eventually returns to playing hockey without symptoms. However, 18 months later the child returns with a complaint of right knee buckling and odd appearance. On exam, the child is now significantly "knock-kneed" on the right. New x-rays show sclerosis and narrowing at the lateral proximal tibial physis but not the medial side, which is clearly patent. In addition, the proximal tibia has grown into valgus. Despite appropriate initial treatment of the fracture, there has been a growth arrest at the lateral proximal tibia. This has resulted in an acquired deformity that will require surgery to correct.

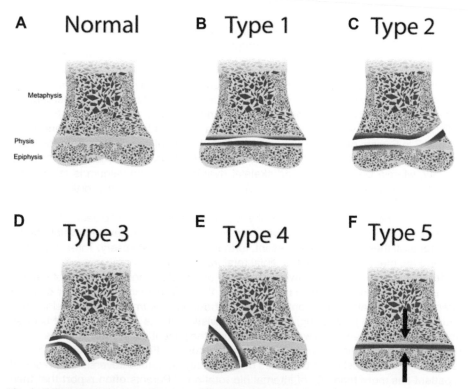

Fig. 1. Salter Harris Fracture Patterns. (Illustrated by Colin Noyes.)

Pearl
Physeal injuries may lead to partial or complete growth arrest and subsequent acquired varus deformity, valgus deformity or limb length difference. Some Salter Harris fractures require monitoring to rule out these long-term sequelae.

Physes are also prone to overuse syndromes. An example is Little League shoulder wherein repetitive throwing can lead to growth plate widening and pain. Another overuse syndrome in the growing child is apophysitis. An apophysis is a secondary ossification center that, unlike an epiphysis, does not constitute part of a joint. In some cases, tendons attach directly to apophyses. These areas can be especially prone to pain in adolescence. Repetitive movement (ie, running, ascending stairs, or jumping) creates the recurrent traction of the tendon on the apophysis leading to soft tissue inflammation and apophyseal fragmentation. Examples include Osgood Schlatter's disease (where the patellar tendon attaches to the tibial tubercle), Sever's disease (where the achilles tendon attaches to the calcaneal apophysis), or Iselin disease (where the peroneal tendon attaches to the apophysis at the base of the fifth metatarsal). Mainstay management for these conditions is non-operative and typically includes icing, stretching, NSAIDs, physical therapy, activity modification, and occasional bracing.[6] While apophysitis are not dangerous, symptoms can be functionally limiting and persistent.

Limb Deformities

Genu varum, genu valgum, and intoeing are common variants in limb alignment. They are typically physiologic and without serious clinical implications. However, clinicians must be familiar with red flag signs and symptoms that necessitate further workup.

Genu varum "bowed legs" is common in children under the age of two and often requires only observation to monitor for progressive resolution.

Pearl
Red flags requiring orthopedic referral include unilateral or asymmetric bowing, lack of improvement by 2 years of age, nutritional deficiencies, short stature (<5th percentile), or family history of pathologic genu varum (such as Blount's disease).[7]

Physiologic genu valgum ("knock-knees") may present in the toddler years, peak around 3 to 5 years of age, and improve by 7 to 8 years of age. Risk factors for pathologic genu valgum include asymmetric deformity, history of infection, prior trauma, obesity, vitamin D deficiency, and skeletal dysplasia. If genu valgum is still prominent or worsening beyond the age of 7, a referral to pediatric orthopedics is appropriate.[8]

A common benign rotational deformity in children is intoeing (or "pigeon-toeing"). In general, intoeing is not associated with pain, limp, or delay in achieving developmental milestones. If these findings are present, further work up is necessary. Three causes of intoeing are metatarsus adductus, tibial torsion, and femoral anteversion.[9]

Metatarsus adductus is an inward curvature of the lateral border of the foot caused by in utero positioning. Parents usually notice this deformity in the first year of life. It often resolves by about 18 months of age without any treatment. Tibial torsion, also caused by in utero positioning, is an inward twisting of one or both tibias. It is often noticed when children begin walking. Evaluating the patient's thigh-foot angle is a simple way to detect either internal or external tibial torsion (**Fig. 2**). Tibial torsion usually resolves spontaneously by 4 to 5 years of age. Lastly, femoral anteversion is present if a patient has more than 60° of internal hip rotation.[10] Parents often report that their child "w-sits." Intoeing from femoral anteversion may improve until the age of 7 to 8.

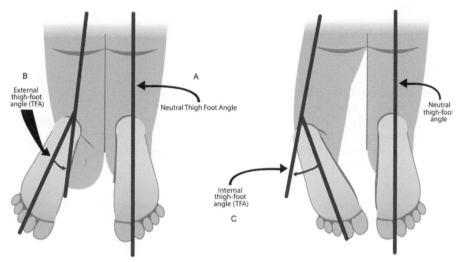

Fig. 2. Evaluation of thigh-foot angle. (Illustrated by Colin Noyes.)

Scoliosis

Scoliosis is a greater than 10-degree lateral curvature and rotation of the spine away from midline. Various subtypes include congenital, idiopathic (infantile, juvenile, adolescent), neuromuscular, and secondary scoliosis (which results from an underlying syndrome or structural lesion). While adolescent idiopathic scoliosis (AIS) is by far the most common subtype, a thorough history and evaluation is imperative to avoid overlooking a non-skeletal etiology.[7] History taking should include.

- Markers of physiologic maturity (growth chart, menses)
- Inquiries of back pain
- Review of neurologic symptoms such as gait abnormality, paresthesia, weakness, changes in bowel or bladder habits
- Family history

Scoliosis typically presents as a concern of asymmetrical appearance of the back or shoulders. Only one-quarter of adolescents with scoliosis present with pain.[8]

Pearl
Significant pain with nighttime waking, functional limitations, or other associated neurologic symptoms indicate the need for further evaluation with x-ray and/or MRI due to concern for cord or nerve root compression.[9]

Physical Exam

Inspection may reveal neurocutaneous markings, shoulder asymmetry or pelvic obliquity. Examination for scoliosis is incomplete without Adams forward bend assessment, described here.

- Patient stands with feet facing forward, knees straight, and palms together.
- Patient bends forward slowly and as far as they can with knees straight
- Looking across the back like a tabletop, check for thoracic or lumbar prominences
- A scoliometer may assist in determining the degree of trunk rotation[10]

Pearl

A scoliometer measurement of less than 5 degrees has a 99% sensitivity and 97% specificity for curves less than 20 degrees and does not typically prompt imaging.[11]

Imaging

An x-ray (AP spine survey) allows for the measurement of scoliotic curves utilizing the Cobb method. One identifies the apex of the curve and proceeds above and below the apex to the most tilted vertebrae. A Cobb angle measures the degree of difference between the long axes of these tilted vertebrae. Scoliotic curves measure greater than 10°. The most common curve pattern in AIS is a dextroconvex (right-sided apex) thoracic curve with a levoconvex (left-sided apex) lumbar curve.

Pearl

*Levoconvex thoracic or dextroconvex lumbar curves are more suggestive of secondary scoliosis and warrant further investigation (*Fig. 3*).*[9]

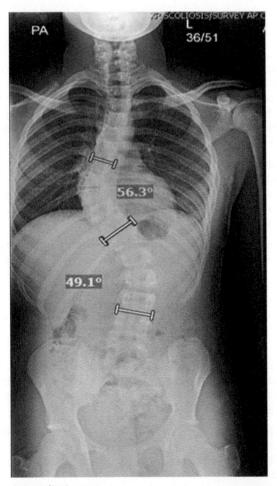

Fig. 3. X-ray measuring scoliotic curve.

Treatment and Prognosis

It is appropriate to refer skeletally immature patients with curves greater than 10° (Cobb angle) to a pediatric orthopedist. Once referred, the specialist will periodically examine the child and obtain x-rays to watch for progression. If a skeletally immature patient's curve progresses beyond 25°, the specialist will likely recommend bracing.

Pearl

The goal of bracing is to prevent curve progression, not to correct the current curvature. Bracing continues until skeletal maturity, at which point curve progression is unlikely. Unfortunately, some curves progress despite bracing. Scoliotic curves that progress to 50° in the thoracic spine or 45° in the lumbar spine warrant surgical intervention because these severe curves can progress despite skeletal maturity.[12] Curves that do not reach surgical range are not associated with functional limitations or pain later in life.

Growing Pains

Up to a third of school-aged children experience growing pains.[13] Providers who care for children are likely to encounter growing pains. While growing pains are extremely common, pediatric orthopedists still do not fully understand the etiology. Because growing pains are a diagnosis of exclusion, providers face the burden of ruling out other less common but important diagnoses.

Pearl

Concerning historical points or physical exam findings warrant further evaluation.[14]

Case #2. *An otherwise healthy 5-year-old female presents with leg pain. Her parents report that she has been waking up at night screaming and complaining of pain in her lower legs. They have tried massage and icing, which sometimes helps. Other times she needs acetaminophen or ibuprofen to fall asleep. When she wakes up the next morning, she is asymptomatic and participating normally in all activities. The evening pain occurs 3 to 4 nights/week. The parents are nervous this may indicate an ominous underlying problem.*

On exam, the child appears well and is playing on the exam table. There is no edema, erythema, or rash. There is age-appropriate tibial bruising. The legs are non-tender save some scant discomfort along the calves. Range of motion in the hips, knees and ankles is full, symmetric, and painless. She hops off the exam table without hesitation, happily jumps about the exam room, and walks with a non-antalgic gait.

Growing pain is a clinical diagnosis with a specific pattern of symptomatology. Later in discussion are some key features/common trends.

- Lower extremity pain presenting in children 2 to 12 years old.
- Often bilateral, but unilateral in 15% of cases
- Pain typically occurs in the late afternoon, evening, or at night, sometimes with nighttime waking.
- Intermittent symptoms resolving by morning with no limping.
- Pain ranges from mild to severe aching
- Massage, heat, or Tylenol/NSAIDs alleviates symptoms
- Clinical exam, x-rays, and laboratory studies are normal
- Symptoms resolve with skeletal maturity[14]

Growing pains are self-limited and do not cause long-term problems. Evaluation with bloodwork and imaging is often unnecessary if a patient presents with typical symptomatology and a normal exam. However, atypical findings warrant further evaluation even if suspicion for growing pains is high. The onus is on the clinician to rule out other causes of bone pain (such as fracture, tumor, infection, or rheumatologic process) before committing to growing pains as the diagnosis. The following are symptoms warranting additional work up.

- Unilateral pain
- Severe pain
- Limping or non-weight bearing
- Point tenderness, redness, swelling, or muscle wasting on exam
- Associated symptoms such as fever, chills, night sweats, poor appetite, unexplained weight loss

Additional work up may include labs (complete blood count, lactate dehydrogenase, C-reactive protein, erythrocyte sedimentation rate) to lower suspicion of infection, malignancy, or inflammatory process, or x-rays to rule out an osseous lesion or fracture.

Developmental Dysplasia of the Hip

DDH is the underdevelopment of the hip joint. While asymptomatic at birth, DDH can cause significant problems for patients later in life. DDH is a "do-not-miss" diagnosis in pediatric orthopedics, but unfortunately it can be easy to overlook. Familiarity with the risk factors and signs of DDH will help prevent delayed diagnosis. Primary risk factors include.

- First born child
- Female sex
- Family history of hip dysplasia–especially in a sibling
- Breech positioning in utero *(PEARL: Breech positioning at any point during the pregnancy–not just delivery–increases the risk of hip dysplasia.)*

Physical exam

Because infants and young children with hip dysplasia are typically asymptomatic, physical exam is critical in diagnosing hip dysplasia. Physical exam findings differ based on the child's age. When examining a newborn, the following maneuvers are most useful.

- Galeazzi maneuver detects a leg length difference if there is a unilateral dislocation
- Barlow maneuver dislocates an unstable hip
- Ortolani maneuver reduces a dislocated hip
- Klisic sign detects the superior displacement of the femur relative to the pelvis, see **Fig. 4**

Pearl

Providers can easily miss bilateral hip dislocations on Galeazzi. The Klisic test is more sensitive in these cases. Abduction: detects stiffness. Will be limited (<60°) or asymmetric (in unilateral dysplasia) in patients older than 3 months.

Pearl

After 2 to 3 months of age, Barlow and Ortolani maneuvers become less reliable as detection tools. At this point, one must rely more heavily on detecting asymmetry on Galeazzi, limited abduction, and gait irregularity.

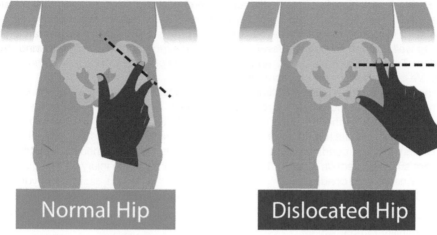

Fig. 4. The Klisic test. (Illustrated by Colin Noyes.)

Diagnosis and referral

If a clinician suspects a diagnosis of hip dysplasia, it is essential to order the appropriate imaging to confirm the diagnosis and/or refer to a specialist. For newborns with positive physical exam findings, one should obtain an ultrasound of both hips with manipulation within a week or two. If the newborn has risk factors but no concerning exam findings, delay the ultrasound until 6 to 8 weeks of age, correcting for prematurity.[15] If you suspect hip dysplasia in a child who is 6 months of age or older, x-rays of the hips (AP and frog lateral of both hips) is the preferred study. Prompt referral to a pediatric orthopedist is appropriate if one suspects hip dysplasia based on risk factors, physical exam findings, or imaging.

Treatment and prognosis

In most cases, orthopedists treat infants with DDH with abduction bracing (either a Pavlik harness or rhino brace). This is often the only necessary treatment, and most children go on to have perfectly functioning, painless hips throughout life. In more severe cases, surgery may be required to relocate the femoral head or reshape the acetabulum. Regardless of severity, children with hip dysplasia require long term monitoring by a specialist.

The Limping Child

Limping is a common presenting symptom that is associated with many diagnoses ranging from a minor sprain to a malignant tumor. Because the causes vary widely, pinpointing an accurate diagnosis can pose a significant challenge.[16] A systematic approach to the evaluation of limping is critical to ensure that one does not overlook a grave condition. In addition to a thorough history and physical exam, understanding which conditions are more common based on the child's age and knowing the appropriate diagnostic tests is critical to establishing a diagnosis. It is not possible to cover all diagnoses associated with limping in this brief section, but the following are useful examples.

Toddlers (1–3 years)

Case #3. *An otherwise healthy 2-year-old toddler presents with progressively worsening pain and guarding of the right leg over the past 24 hours. They will not walk* *on their own and the family recently noticed redness and swelling around the right knee. Any time the caregivers try to move the patient's right knee, the child cries. The child has been more irritable since the symptoms began and is not sleeping or eating well. Caregivers report a fever of 101.8 F this morning for which they gave the patient Tylenol. Given the fever, refusal to bear weight and severity of symptoms, you are concerned for an infectious process.*

The most common causes of limp in a toddler include transient synovitis, septic arthritis, discitis, toddler's fracture, cerebral palsy, muscular dystrophy, developmental dysplasia of the hip, coxa vara, juvenile arthritis, leukemia, and osteoid osteoma.[17] When evaluating a limp or painful lower extremity in a toddler, the clinician must first exclude conditions that could have serious and/or immediate deleterious impact such as infection (septic arthritis or osteomyelitis), acute injury, oncologic process or neurologic condition.

Red flags associated with a limp in a toddler include.

- Fever
- Inability to bear weight
- Redness or swelling
- Child appearing unwell or toxic
- Recent unintentional weight loss
- Regression of motor milestones
- Findings concerning for non-accidental trauma[17]

If a child presents with any of these red flag symptoms in conjunction with a limp, referral to an emergency department is appropriate. Immediate work up should include x-rays and bloodwork (complete blood count with differential, C-reactive protein, erythrocyte sedimentation rate ± blood cultures, Lyme titers and creatinine kinase).

Kocher's criteria is a helpful tool used to predict the likelihood of septic arthritis in the hip. The criteria include four independent clinical predictors: history of associated fever, inability to bear weight, erythrocyte sedimentation rate of at least 40 mm/hr, and white blood cell count of 12,000 cells/mL. The probability of septic arthritis in the presence of these factors is as follows.

- 0/4 predictive factors: <0.2%
- 1/4 predictive factors: 3.0%
- 2/4 predictive factors: 40.0%
- 3/4 predictive factors: 93.1%
- 4/4 predictive factors: 99.6%[17]

Kocher's criteria are helpful in determining whether a limp requires immediate referral to the emergency department or simply close observation and follow up.

Pearl

If a toddler is well-appearing, afebrile, bearing weight on the extremity, eating, and drinking well, and has no visible redness or swelling, emergent referral is likely unnecessary.

School age (4–10 years)

The most common causes of limp in the school age population include transient synovitis, septic arthritis, Legg-Calve-Perthes disease, discoid meniscus, and limb length discrepancy.[17] Other causes are possible, including those mentioned in the toddler section.

Case #4. *A 7-year-old developmentally typical child with no significant past medical or surgical history presents for the evaluation of a new painful limp and intermittent unwillingness to bear weight on the left leg. The child had a viral upper respiratory infection 3 weeks ago, but symptoms have fully resolved. There is no history of trauma. The child was asymptomatic when they went to bed and awoke with symptoms. The child ate a typical breakfast and is otherwise well with no associated fever, malaise, weight loss, or fatigue. Caregivers administered Motrin, which seemed to improve symptoms. The child does not complain of pain at rest, but when they try to walk, they indicate pain around the right hip. On exam, there is no redness, swelling or deformity of the lower extremity. There is some discomfort and limitation with the passive motion of the hip. There is no point tenderness. Gait is antalgic. Based on your history and exam you are suspicious for transient synovitis.*

Transient or toxic synovitis is the most common cause of limp in children 3 to 8 years of age. It presents as joint irritation, often in the setting of antecedent viral illness.[17] This condition is a diagnosis of exclusion. Because transient synovitis mimics septic arthritis or osteomyelitis, x-rays of the hip, blood work, and joint aspiration are often necessary but will likely yield normal results. Typically, symptoms resolve in 1 to 2 weeks. Treatment is symptomatic and includes activity modification, limited or restricted weight bearing, and use of NSAIDs. Outcomes are very favorable.

Adolescent (11–15)
The most common causes of limping in adolescence include slipped capital femoral epiphysis (SCFE), hip dysplasia, chondrolysis, overuse syndromes, and osteochondritis dissecans.[17]

Case #5. *A 12-year-old male with a BMI of 32 and no relevant past medical history presents with 1 month of atraumatic left knee pain. He has a history of mild asthma, but otherwise has no significant past medical or surgical history. his pediatrician suggested conditioning and weight loss to improve symptoms. He wanted to play football but was not able to run and keep up with his peers due to knee pain. He denies redness or swelling. His mother notices a limp and reports "he walks funny now," but he is only minimally aware of this.*

Knee exam is negative for redness, swelling, tenderness or joint instability. He has full and unrestricted ROM. On supine exam, he is noted to have a leg length discrepancy of approximately 2 cm, left shorter than right. Hip ROM reveals obligatory external rotation and abduction on the left. Left internal hip rotation is significantly limited and provokes pain; there are 30 degrees of internal rotation on the right. You order x-rays of the patient's hips (bilateral, AP and frog-lateral). This is confusing to the patient and family, as his complaint is the left knee. You explain your concern for Slipped-Capital Femoral Epiphysis (SCFE) and proceed.

SCFE occurs when the capital femoral epiphysis displaces, typically posterior and medial displacement, on the femoral neck. SCFE occurs most commonly at ages 12 to 15 in boys and 10 to 13 in girls. Risk factors include obesity, male sex, endocrine disorders, and femoral retroversion. The slippage can occur gradually or acutely and is categorized as stable (able to bear weight) or unstable (unable to bear weight). Typical symptoms include hip pain, groin pain, asymmetric gait, or knee pain.

Pearl
SCFE may present with only knee pain, as the obturator nerve can be irritated from slippage. Therefore, always examine the hips in older children presenting with knee pain. Exam findings often include pain with the mobilization of hip, asymmetric gait, leg length discrepancy, and obligatory external rotation with flexion of affected hip and

absence of any internal rotation. X-rays (AP and frog-lateral views) confirm the diagnosis. An acute and unstable SCFE should warrant immediate referral to an emergency department while a chronic stable SCFE can be seen urgently by an orthopedic surgeon within 1 to 2 days. Treatment involves percutaneous fixation. Even with appropriate referral and intervention, there is a risk of avascular necrosis of the femoral head (up to 47% in unstable SCFE) and limited range of motion.[17]

SUMMARY

Pediatric orthopedics is a unique subspecialty that relies on an understanding of the developing skeleton and physiologic norms from infancy to adolescence. This knowledge paired with thorough history-taking and honed physical exam skills leads to prompt diagnosis, timely treatment, and prevention of future complications. This fundamental review has highlighted some "do not miss" and "high-yield" topics that clinicians are likely to encounter when treating children with orthopedic complaints. It has hopefully served to both excite the budding orthopedic provider about the unique qualities of the pediatric skeleton and to remind clinicians that a thorough history and physical exam are key to assigning the correct diagnosis.

CLINICS CARE POINTS

- The pediatric skeleton is unique in terms of ossification, remodeling potential, and the presence of growth plates
- Physeal injuries are common; some can lead to growth arrest and progressive deformity
- Genu varum, genu valgum, and intoeing are often physiologic, but clinicians must consider pathologic causes
- Growing pains are a diagnosis of exclusion
- All pediatric generalists should be comfortable evaluating for scoliosis and hip dysplasia and know when to refer
- There are many causes of limping in children that range from benign to serious. It is essential to rule out dangerous diagnoses first.
- Asymmetry (in appearance, motion, function, and so forth) is often cause for concern
- Always assess the joint above and below the level of complaint
- Be familiar with red flag signs and symptoms that may arise with history taking and raise suspicion for ominous diagnoses.
- Consider NAT when history and exam are incongruent

DISCLOSURE

The authors have nothing to disclose.

REFERENCES

1. Paul AR, Adamo MA. Non-accidental trauma in pediatric patients: a review of epidemiology, pathophysiology, diagnosis and treatment. Transl Pediatr 2014; 3(3):195–207.
2. Sponseller PD. Anatomy and Normal Development in Children. In: Handbook of pediatric orthopaedics. 3rd edition. New York, NY: Thieme; 2020. p. 9–13.

3. Kecler-Pietrzyk A, Normal elbow, radius and ulna x-ray - 6-year-old. Case study, Radiopaedia.org (Accessed on 07 Apr 2023) https://doi.org/10.53347/rID-53556.

4. Diab M. Trauma. In: Staheli LA, editor. Practice of paediatric orthopaedics. 3rd edition. Philadelphia, PA: Wolters Kluwer; 2016. p. 136–8.

5. Wimberly RL. General Principles of Managing Orthopaedic Injuries. In: Herring JA, editor. Tachdjian's pediatric orthopaedics : from the Texas scottish rite hospital for children. 6th edition. Philadelphia, PA: Elsevier; 2022. p. 1131–55. Available at: https://www.clinicalkey.com/#!/content/book/3-s2.0-B9780323567695000272?scrollTo=%23top. Accessed April 5, 2023.

6. Beck J. Osgood-Schlatter. Available at: https://posna.org/physician-education/study-guide/osgood-schlatter. Accessed March 30, 2023.

7. Janicki JA, Alman B. Scoliosis: Review of diagnosis and treatment. Paediatr Child Health 2007;12(9):771–6.

8. Ramirez N, Johnston C, Browne RH. The prevalence of back pain in children who have idiopathic scoliosis. J Bone Joint Surg 1997;79(3):364–8.

9. Society SR. Scoliosis Research Society. Professional Online Education: Conditions and Treatments.- Available at: https://www.srs.org/professionals/online-education-and-resources/conditions-and-treatments. Published 2023. Accessed March 31, 2023.

10. Horne JP, Flannery R, Usman S. Adolescent Idiopathic Scoliosis: Diagnosis and Management. Am Fam Physician 2014;89(3):193–8.

11. Sponseller PD. Disorders of Spinal Growth and DevelopmentPa. In: Handbook of pediatric orthopaedics. New York, NY: Thieme; 2020. p. 109–23.

12. Society SR. Available at: Scoliosis Research Society. Professional Online Education: Conditions and Treatments.- https://www.srs.org/professionals/online-education-and-resources/conditions-and-treatments. Published 2023. Accessed March 31, 2023.

13. Junnila JL, Cartwright VW. Chronic Musculoskeletal Pain in Children: Part I. Initial Evaluation Am Fam Physician 2006;74(1):115–22.

14. Cappello T. Growing Pains. Available at: https://posna.org/physician-education/study-guide/growingpains. Accessed March 23, 2023.

15. Kim HKW, Herring JA. Developmental Dysplasia of the Hip. In: Tachdjian's pediatric orthopaedics : from the Texas scottish rite hospital for children. Vol 2. 6th edition. Philadelphia, PA: Elsevier; 2022. p. 422–526. Available at: https://search.library.yale.edu/catalog/15914777. Accessed April 5, 2023.

16. Staheli LT. Fundamentals of pediatric orthopedics. 4th edition. Philadelphia, PA: Lippincott, Williams & Wilkins; 2008. p. 136.

17. Herring JA, Birch JG. The Limping Child. In: Herring JA, editor. Tachdjian's pediatric:from the Texas scottish rite hospital for children. 5th edition. Philadelphia, PA: Elsevier Saunders; 2014. p. 80–7.

Becoming Whole Again
How Prosthetics Shape the Human Experience

Alexander Hopkins, MSPA, PA-C[a],*,
Rodney Ho, MPAS, MPH, PhD, PA-C, Psychiatry-CAQ[b],
Derrick Varner, PhD, PA-C, DFAAPA, RDMS[c]

KEYWORDS

• Prosthetics • Military • Veteran • Orthotics • Physical therapy

KEY POINTS

• Discuss the history of prosthetics.
• Explore how prosthetics became a necessity.
• Describe the psychological impact of limb, eye loss, and replacement.
• Look forward to the future of prosthetic use.

INTRODUCTION

As long as humans have existed, the possibility of limb loss has accompanied them. Absent the ability to grow these appendages back, a person was left stricken for life—the remainder of which was often terribly short. This begged the invention of replacement parts for the unfortunate. Whether functional or cosmetic, prosthetics predate the Common Era, demonstrating a long, beneficial, and currently prospering area of medical care.

Prosthetics taken as a field is remarkably broad. It can encompass aids to help with activities of daily living, implanted devices such as mechanical knees, hips, or they can be palliative devices such as knee braces. They may even be monitoring devices like automatic sphygmomanometers for home use.

For the sake of brevity and an appreciation toward capturing the most considered clinical applications, this article will focus on prosthetics replacing the arms, legs, eyes, and hands. Additionally, the article will focus on applications in the veteran population. Unfortunately, modern warfare is likely to deprive veterans of limb and eyesight.

HISTORY

A woman in Cairo, Egypt,[1] lost a part of herself between 950 and 700 BCE. This inspired the earliest known prosthetic. As human technology is often wont, this early

[a] Physician Assistant, Orlando VA Medical Center, Viera Outpatient Clinic, 2900 Veterans Way, Melbourne, FL 32940, USA; [b] Rocky Mountain University; [c] Family Medicine
* Corresponding author.
E-mail address: Al321hopkins@gmail.com

Physician Assist Clin 9 (2024) 137–147
https://doi.org/10.1016/j.cpha.2023.08.004
2405-7991/24/Published by Elsevier Inc.

physicianassistant.theclinics.com

prosthetic was as humble as it comes: a right great toe. The Cairo Toe, as it came to be called, was made of wood with a leather adapter allowing it to be attached to the foot. Small leather straps were provided for adjustment. It was found on the mummy of an Egyptian noblewoman, presumably one of the elites who could afford a craftsman.

History knows of no other prosthetics until 100 years later when the circa 600 BCE Greville Chester toe was discovered. This is another Egyptian invention, discovered in 2000 near Luxor.[2]

It would be another 300 years before any advancements were made. The Capua leg was discovered in 1910.[3] Made of bronze and plaster and excavated from an ancient grave in Capua, Italy, it is the oldest known example of an artificial limb. Regrettably, the original limb was in London in World War II and was destroyed in a bombing raid. **Fig. 1** is a picture of a replica leg currently held with the Royal College of Surgeons, England.

After the common era in circa 476 to 1000 (the Middle Ages), the archetypal peg leg and hand hooks came to be. As with the Cairo toe, fitment of these prosthetics was reserved for those who could afford it. For example, knights could be fitted with devices to hold shields or help them mount horses. These assistive devices were tailor made by craftsman (which explains the cost) and were increasingly complex. Some could even use gears and springs.

This trend continued through the renaissance where most prosthetics were made from copper, iron, steel, and wood. **Fig. 2** is an excellent example of the limbs of this time. It belonged to Gottfried "Götz" von Berlichingen, a famed mercenary from the 1500s. Götz was assisting in the invasion of Landshut in 1504 when an enemy cannon was fired. The projectile struck a blade he was holding, forcing it backward on to his right arm.[4] German doctors deemed the limb beyond salvage, and he underwent amputation of the right wrist and hand. Unwilling to put his military career to an end, Götz twice commissioned blacksmiths to fashion him an iron right wrist and hand. The engineering of the limb is quite impressive, particularly in the second model. His chief requirement was being able to use a sword. The original iron hand used 4 fingers and a system of hinges that would flex the digits in pairs of 2. A button on the wrist would spring them back to an extended position.

The complexity and functionality markedly increased in the second model seen in **Fig. 3**. The degree of biomimicry was unprecedented. Digits 2 through 4 had three hinges to reflect the metacarpophalangeal, proximal interphalangeal, and distal interphalangeal joints. Digit one had 2 joints, analogous to the thumb. The digits could be flexed and locked in place. As with the first model, buttons were used to extend the

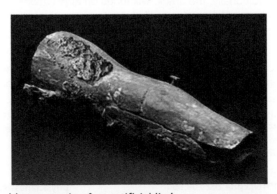

Fig. 1. Replica of oldest example of an artificial limb.

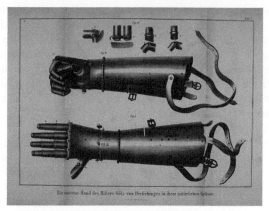

Fig. 2. Example of a prosthetic from Renaissance period.

spring-loaded fingers. Additionally, the wrist could be angled multiple ways to allow for gripping reins, using a sword, and even using a feather pen.

This served him for 15 years and earned him the nickname "Götz of the iron hand." His story is deeply woven into Renaissance folklore. Around 200 years after his death, Johann Wolfgang von Goethe wrote a play based on his life.[5] He is also featured on plaques with his famous off-color quote in response to a call to surrender during battle (**Fig. 3**).

The civil war arguably began the modern era of prosthetics, particularly where veterans are concerned. There were an estimated 60,000 amputations from both the North and the South and 75% of these patients survived.[6]

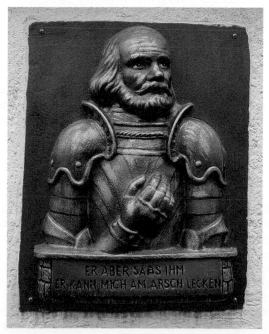

Fig. 3. Plaque of Gottfried "Götz" von Berlichingen. Götz von Berlichingen in Weisenheim am Sand, Germany. Immanuel Giel. https://commons.wikimedia.org/wiki/File:Goetz_von_Berlichingen_in_Weisenheim_am_Sand.jpg.

Owing to the en-masse field formations and use of blunt projectiles, the Civil War was a truly brutal conflict. Not only were limbs lost, but eyes and pieces of skull. This led to some of the earliest cosmetic procedures. Eyes could be fashioned from glass. In many cases a sphere of charred bone was introduced into the orbital socket with the eyelids sewn shut, the bone providing volume.[7] Additionally, biomimicry of prosthetic joints advanced with articulated lower limbs and rubber hands. Prosthetics also became democratized as the federal government began to issue stipends for soldiers to buy artificial limbs. Patients no longer needed the wealth to hire craftsman or the engineering skill to build their own limbs.

The need to subsidize medical care for wounded veterans led to the National Home for Disabled Soldiers and Sailors in 1865.[8] This is the first government home for honorably discharged veterans. This was in keeping with Abraham Lincoln's promise "To care for him who shall have borne the battle and for his widow, and his orphan."

Through the Civil War and following World Wars, artificial limbs were constrained by the material science of the time—meaning most would still be made of leather and wood. This unfortunately, allowed for the absorption of dirt and sweat. One could only imagine the discomfort, difficulty in cleaning, and odor of these materials.

Material science advancements would usher in a new era of prosthetics. Plastics, resins, polycarbonates, carbon fiber, and laminates became the standard. Not only could the limbs be lighter weight, but they were easier to clean, more customizable, more comfortable, and could be paired with synthetic sockets.[2]

These synthetic materials can withstand the constant physical stress of athletics with no breaking down. Additionally, they lack a porous nature, making sweat easy to clean and providing no harbor for malodorous bacteria.

In the 21st century the pace of development continues to accelerate. Artificial limbs can have small motors and sensors to move automatically. Brain–computer interfaces are being researched, and 3-D printing may revolutionize manufacturing.

BACKGROUND

As is likely gleaned from above, the primary driver of prosthetics advancement was warfare. The Civil War in particular drove prosthetics use owing to the increased availability to purchase limbs through federal government subsidy. This trend continued with the establishment of the Department of Veterans Affairs and its role in medical care in every major conflict since the establishment of the National Home.

To understand the reason for prosthetics, the weapons must be understood. The civil war kicked off the era of government subsidized prosthetics, so it would make sense to begin with that conflict.

Civil war tactics were Napoleonic. Large armies stood in massed formations, each hoping to outlast the other. Sustaining attrition was a key factor in victory.

Unfortunately for the soldiers in those formations, the weapons were imprecise with extreme blunt force. Loss of limb due to cannon fire is self-explanatory, but the weapon of greatest importance may be the Minié ball.

Invented by Claude-Étienne Minié in 1847, its lethality, accuracy compared with musket balls, ease of use, ease of production, and increased accuracy quickly made it the standard round of 19th century warfare.

Fig. 4 is a picture of this projectile. The conical shape pierced the body more readily than a musket ball. The grooves of the round and indentation allowed for more efficient gas buildup behind for increased muzzle velocity and accuracy.

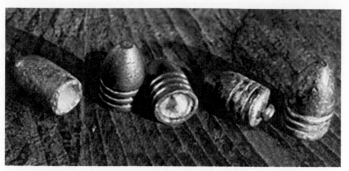

Fig. 4. The Minié ball. Minie Balls, Mike Cumpston. https://commons.wikimedia.org/wiki/File:Minie_Balls.jpg.

The results of Minié ball use did not disappoint field commanders. **Fig. 5** is a femoral head nearly torn off by a rifle using this ammunition. **Fig. 6** is a portrait of a soldier wounded in the arm, necessitating amputation. Both pictures are from the height of the Civil War in 1863.

As a direct result of the Minié ball, amputation became the most common surgical procedure for Union soldiers in the Civil War.[9] Walt Whitman aptly captured the humanity of medicine in the Civil War in his poem The Wound Dresser.[9] In this poem he describes performing wound care on soldiers who will not look at amputated limbs,

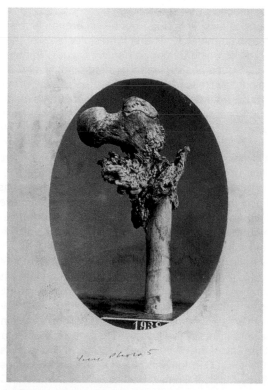

Fig. 5. Picture of a femoral head damaged by the Minié ball. Otis Historical Archives of "National Museum of Health & Medicine" (OTIS Archive 1). https://www.flickr.com/photos/medicalmuseum/4812404941/in/photostream.

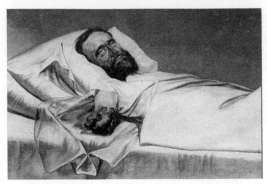

Fig. 6. Portrait of a wounded soldier requiring amputation. Milton Wallen, CWMI098C, National Museum of Health and Medicine. https://www.flickr.com/photos/medicalmuseum/373561781/.

others dying from sepsis, and the emotional stress of working in the field hospitals. **Fig. 7** also depicts a typical scene for Mr Whitman.

World War I would see few improvements in either battlefield tactics or medical care. Yet owing to increased manufacturing capability of warring nations, the brutality was worse.

The industrial revolution saw the dawn of artillery, the machine gun, and combat use of barbed wire. There were countless means of breaking the skin barrier and many means of promoting infection.

Sanitation was poor, and soldiers dug trenches in French farmland which had previously been fertilized with manure.[9] The chief disinfectants of the time were iodine and carbolic acid, both of which damaged healthy tissue. Although harmful bacteria may have been killed, wound healing was therefore complicated.

While soldiers did not have to face the Minié ball, the specter of infection was a constant companion. To be wounded in the trenches meant an almost certain infection. Given the poor wound care techniques, inoculation with fecal coliform among other pathogens, gangrene was common. So too were the amputations to treat it.

The remainder of the 20th century would largely preserve the arms of World War I, but advancements in infection control and the introduction of forward surgical squads greatly increased limb preservation and the survivability of combat.

Instead of care in the field or in a primitive tent hospital, echelons of care evolved from World War II and the Korean war. American wounded receive immediate care and triage in the field from the combat medic. The invention of helicopters allowed for an unprecedented speed of evacuation from the battlefield. These are known as DUSTOFF flights and will often fly under that callsign.

From there, the patient would present to the Battalion Aid Station for simple wounds. This is level I.[9] Level II is the more complicated patient who will initially see the forward resuscitative surgical squad/shock trauma platoon (FRSS/STP.)

A patient needing amputation will receive initial stabilization at the level II FRSS/STP. Ideally, these patients are transported and arrive via helicopter within an hour of injury. For further care, the level III facility is available. These are in theater facilities with intensive care ability. At the end of the chain is level IV, regional hospitals such as Landstuhl Regional Medical Center in Germany and level V, the United States-based hospitals like Walter Reed Army Medical Center, Bethesda Naval Medical Center, and Naval Medical Center Balboa on the west coast.

It would also bear mentioning naval capability via hospital ships like the USNS Comfort and USNS Mercy that provide an additional layer of care. Each of these ships have one thousand beds and surgical capability. These ships further reduce the interval between battlefield injury and evaluation by a surgical squad.

With these complex medical apparatuses in place, it is easily seen why combat survivability in the late 20th and early 21st centuries are beyond comparison to earlier systems before the Vietnam War. Not only will a troop requiring amputation have an increased chance of survival, but prosthetic fitting and rehabilitation will be performed at the level V facility.

It is with these systems in place that history arrives at the most recent conflicts. The Global War on Terror (GWOT) brought new threats to the battlefield. Poorly funded and trained combatants with no centralized structure were pitted against Western-style armed forces.

This necessitated guerilla tactics and improvisation. The improvised explosive device was a weapon of choice. Often made from Soviet and Iraqi surplus munitions, these devices were omnipresent during this conflict. They could be vehicle borne, roadside, or installed on a person. A patrol could be caught unaware with munitions activated by a cellphone, the large blast often causing arm and/or leg amputations, as well as soft tissue injuries depriving eyesight, the latter of which was largely obviated when ballistic goggles became common issue.

Advancements in personal body armor meant the vital organs were shielded, leaving the limbs and hemicranium exposed. This led to amputation being dubbed the signature war wound of the GWOT along with traumatic brain injury.[10]

Fig. 7 illustrates the described protective gear. Ballistic goggles (not seen, but are present) overlie a Kevlar helmet. The modular tactical vest affords protection to the carotid arteries. Unseen is a ceramic insert in the front and back of the Kevlar vest providing robust protection to vital organs. Note the limbs are protected only by fabric, however.

Given the multiple levels of care, modern surgical capability, and modern body armor improving combat survivability, the risk for amputation has decreased since the late 20th and early 21st. However, in the event of an amputation, the options for restoration are more accessible and reliable.

Psychosocial Implications

Loss of a limb affects all aspects of an individual's life and the new physical disability causes psychological and psychosocial problems.[11] The amputee, from the onset of the loss of limb to return to normal life in the community, is beset with doubts and fears. The individual grieves for the limb and old body image. A loss of a limb is a 3 pronged loss in terms of function, sensation, and body image. There is a direct correlation between body image and psychological adjustment and may result in depression, anxiety, and low self-efficacy.

Therefore, it is important to initiate a holistic approach to include psychosocial intervention from onset of loss to the fitting of prosthesis and physical rehabilitation. The fitting of a prosthesis confronts patient with this new reality of having a lost limb. The patient must also contend with learning to be proficient with the new prosthesis. Patients must make permanent behavioral, emotional, and social adjustments to cope with the multitude of problems associated with a loss of limb.[11] There is little attention paid to this subgroup of disabled persons and to the sustained loss of psychological being related to the lost limb and their prosthetic journey to regain physical function. According to Gallagher and McLachlan, incidence of clinical depression among patients with prosthesis in an outpatient setting is common.[11] Patients who are dissatisfied with their prosthesis may manifest as denial or the inability to cope with the prothesis. Patients who have fewer problems with prosthesis itself tend to have fewer emotional problems and exhibit better social integration.

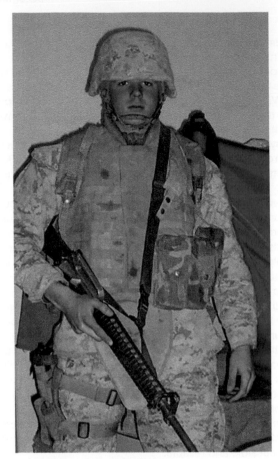

Fig. 7. Protective gear used for personal body armor.

Prolonged pain can impair general function, ability to work, and can cause social and emotional adjustments. Pain specific to the loss of limb refers to phantom limb pain (PLP) and is defined as the sensation of presence of the previous amputated limb. PLP is different for each patient and vary from mild-to-extreme to intermittent or constant pain. PLP is distinguishable from stump pain, which is pain directly at the site of extremity amputation. Those with PLP show a greater degree of despair and withdrawal. However, the phantom limb is believed to be a healthy psychological response due to enhanced proprioceptive feedback that aids in learning to walk.[10] The adjustment of wearing a prothesis varies depending on age, gender, and length of time with prothesis and the cause, degree of disability, and disfigurement at the site of prosthesis. The greatest challenge for young adults with prosthesis is identity and social acceptance. Conversely, older adults contend with ill health, social isolation, psychological resiliency, and financial constraints which may complicate the prosthesis adjustment process. It is important to consider that patients who abandoned their prothesis may repeatedly try several prothesis and continually say it does not fit. A possible mediator for this psychological adjustment is early psychosocial intervention to provide the patient with helpful coping strategies and assist with an increased sense of personal independence and social integration.

Integrating mental health treatment from the onset of limb loss and throughout the process is vital for emotional and mental health wellness. Amputation due to trauma is accompanied by shock, as the individual is unprepared for the loss and experiences greater coping and adaptation difficulties.[12] Amputation-related trauma can increase a person's risk of acute stress reaction, post-traumatic stress syndrome or post-traumatic stress disorder. Mental health professionals can improve psychological and emotional adaptation by normalizing the patient's experience and feelings related to amputation and help the patient utilize adaptive coping mechanisms.[12] In the early stages of rehabilitation, motivational enhancement and solution-focused brief therapy creates a foundation for motivation to change and instill confidence to set and accomplish rehabilitation goals. Acceptance and commitment therapy (ACT) delivered in the middle-to-late stages of rehabilitation is helpful in modifying maladaptive cognitions and mitigate emotional problems caused by change in the treatment process.[12] ACT increases psychological flexibility and adaptation by taking a mindfulness strategy approach that allows the patient to recognize and accept present experiences without judging them. ACT is known to be an effective psychosocial intervention for those suffering from PLP or residual pain and has been shown to be effective in the treatment of associated chronic pain. Cognitive behavioral therapy (CBT) is another effective form of psychological treatment that works by enhancing the patients understanding between thoughts and emotion and how it affects behavior and maladaptive patterns. CBT mediates cognitive restricting and can expand a patient's perspective, enhance cognitive flexibility and assist with modifying automatic thoughts related to amputation and the use of prosthesis. Mindfulness meditation is effective in reducing pain perception, and increases acceptance in patients with anxiety, depression, cancer, and improves overall life satisfaction.

Psychological treatment if delivered early, beginning with amputation or loss of limb, can enhance mental health and emotional wellness. It can prevent co-occurring depression, anxiety, and emotional problems. There are several psychological treatments such as mindfulness mediation, ACT, solution focused brief therapy, and CBT that can assist the patient through all stages of the treatment process to be psychological flexible and modify negative thoughts associated with loss of limb and rehabilitation. The psychological wellness of a patient is just as important as the physical rehabilitation and integrating mental health professionals early in treatment can ease depression, anxiety, chronic pain, and PLP.

DISCUSSION

The first use of a prosthetic is dated back to the Common Era. Since then, there have been many advancements due to research and technology. Since the late 20th century, the military has created processes to help decrease the number of amputations caused by warfare. These processes, along with the research done to improve prosthetics have radically changed the physical outcomes of patients that undergo amputations. The mental and emotional outcomes of these patients have also been researched and it demonstrates that psychological intervention affects physical outcomes. Therefore, it is important that the mental and emotional well-being of patients with amputations be addressed at the onset of loss for increasing the likelihood of the patient becoming and feeling whole again.

CLINICS CARE POINTS

- Patients experience loss of limb from various causes including warfare, exposure to chemicals, and chronic diseases.

- Psychological impacts affect patients from the moment they experience the loss of limb and continue into the rehabilitation and prosthetic fitting phase.
- Early psychological treatment can enhance mental and emotional wellness.
- The physical restoration of a lost limb with a prosthetic and the mental and emotional treatment of experiencing the loss go hand in hand in making the patient whole again.

DISCLOSURE

The author has no financial or personal conflicts of interest in this subject. Images used are in public domain and not subject to copywrite.

REFERENCES

1. Garber, M. (2013, November 21). The perfect, 3,000-year-old toe: A brief history of prosthetic limbs. The Atlantic. Retrieved March 3, 2023, from https://www.theat lantic.com/technology/archive/2013/11/the-perfect-3-000-year-old-toe-a-brief-history-of-prosthetic-limbs/281653/.
2. Admin, U. P. M. C. (2020, February 7). Timeline: Prosthetic limbs through the years. UPMC HealthBeat. Retrieved March 8, 2023, from https://share.upmc.com/2015/03/timeline-prosthetic-limbs-years/.
3. Royal College of Surgeons, England. (n.d.). Copy of roman artificial leg, London, England, 1905-1915: Science Museum Group Collection. Copy of Roman artificial leg, London, England, 1905-1915 | Science Museum Group. Retrieved March 21, 2023, from https://collection.sciencemuseumgroup.org.uk/objects/co84549/copy-of-roman-artificial-leg-london-england-1905-1915-artificial-leg.
4. Ashmore K, Cialdella S, Giuffrida A, et al. ArtiFacts: Gottfried "Götz" von Berlichingen-The "Iron Hand" of the Renaissance. Clin Orthop Relat Res 2019;477(9):2002–4.
5. von Goethe, J. (2012, July 24). Goetz of Berlichingen, with the iron hand. Google Books. Retrieved March 23, 2023, from https://books.google.com/books?hl=en&lr=&id=bE5SAAAAcAAJ&oi=fnd&pg=PP3&ots=J4Jket1mZA&sig=oVQAnBj Wt24ARnsGYwL0Obdh87o#v=onepage&q&f=false.
6. Labbe, S. (2018, March 16). Inspirations of war: Innovations in prosthetics after the Civil War. Inspirations of War: Innovations in Prosthetics after the Civil War. Retrieved March 23, 2023, from https://cupola.gettysburg.edu/cgi/viewcontent. cgi?article=1361&context=compiler.
7. Hughes, M. (n.d.). Eye injuries and prosthetic restoration in the American Civil War Years. Journal of Ophthalmic Prosthetics. Retrieved March 23, 2023, from http://wordpress.artificialeyeclinic.com/wp-content/uploads/2015/06/civilwar.pdf.
8. U.S. Department of Veterans Affairs. (2022, November 1). History overview. U.S. Department of Veterans Affairs. Retrieved March 23, 2023, from https://department.va.gov/history/history-overview/.
9. Manring, M. M., Hawk, A., Calhoun, J. H., & Andersen, R. C. (2009, August). Treatment of war wounds: A historical review. Clinical orthopaedics and related research. Retrieved March 28, 2023, from https://www.ncbi.nlm.nih.gov/pmc/articles/PMC2706344/.
10. Wallace, D., (2022, November 15) Trends in traumatic limb amputation in Allied forces in Iraq and Afghanistan. JMVH. Retrieved April 13, 2023, from https://jmvh.org/article/trends-in-traumatic-limb-amputation-in-allied-forces-in-iraq-and-afghanistan/.

11. Gallagher P, MacLachlan M. Psychological adjustment and coping in adults with prosthetic limbs. Behav Med 1999;25(3):117–24. https://doi.org/10.1080/089642 89909596741.

12. Wang Y et al., "Effective Evaluation of Finger Sensation Evoking by Non-Invasive Stimulation for Sensory Function Recovery in Transradial Amputees," in IEEE Transactions on Neural Systems and Rehabilitation Engineering, vol. 30, pp. 519-528, 2022, doi: 10.1109/TNSRE.2022.3155756.

The Future of Orthopedics
Imagining Orthopedics in the Year 2100

Courtney L. Bennett Wilke, MPAS, PA-C, Brittany M. Dowdle, BA*

KEYWORDS

- Future of orthopedics • Nanomedicine • Nanobiomechanics • Gene therapy • 3D
- Artificial intelligence • AI

KEY POINTS

- Global health outcomes can be improved through the responsible use of advanced technology, particularly in orthopedics.
- By harnessing new technologies, cost-effective, health-maintaining care can become standard and accessible to all populations.
- In the future, medicine can be more patient-centered and more successful at preventing disease while featuring less invasive, side-effect-prone interventions.

AN ORTHOPEDICS 101 CLASSROOM IN THE YEAR 2100

The professor called the class to attention. He cleared his throat, pausing for dramatic effect.

"How did they practice medicine in the early twenty-first century? At the time, medicine was a rudimentary science at best. It was based on simple facts, cause and effect—almost a study in straightforward mechanics, if you will. Practitioners of the day had a very limited understanding of the power of what we might call *nuanced manipulation*."

"Professor Wendt," called one student. "I don't understand. How can you say that their practice was rudimentary? It sounds as though you are suggesting it was formulaic."

"Indeed, I am proposing that it was exactly that—formulaic!" The professor warmed to his topic, rubbing his hands together. "Take orthopedics, for example. In no other field are the advancements in medicine better illustrated. Think of how they used to treat arthritis, overuse injuries, traumatic fractures—twenty-first-century orthopedists could be considered simple mechanics of the human body, and indeed, in looking back, that is exactly what they were. Think of our trauma patients! Imagine a time when metallic screws were driven into the bone to stabilize shattered limbs—how does this differ from basic carpentry?

Tallahassee Memorial Hospital, 2001, Atapha Nene, Tallahassee, FL 32301, USA
* Corresponding author.
E-mail address: brittany@wordcat-editorial.com

Physician Assist Clin 9 (2024) 149–153
https://doi.org/10.1016/j.cpha.2023.09.002
2405-7991/24/© 2023 Elsevier Inc. All rights reserved.

"In that period, when a patient's joint had been ravaged by time and overuse, imagine—they used to physically cut out the joint and replace it with a standard out-of-the-box replacement! The very thought gives me chills! After decades of this approach, their most significant progress involved custom 3D-printed joints, which, granted, were much more effective at addressing a patient's pain and immobility. And yet how limited is that approach—to wait until the body fails before implementing a plan to treat it!"

"Today, with our understanding of the progression of joint aging and the monitoring afforded by our AI-enabled nanomedicine, we can not only detect microtrauma years in advance of any physically identifiable damage but we are able to deploy preventive technologies to avoid the destruction of the joint in the first place. In the twenty-first century, they would have gaped at the idea that we could stop disease progression before it could rightfully be said to have started."

ORTHOPEDICS THEN AND NOW

Despite Professor Wendt's obvious disdain for twenty-first-century medicine, the fact is that from the time that the term *orthopedics* was first used in 1741 until today, the treatment of disease and injury in the musculoskeletal system has undergone a revolutionary change. Although the field started as a study of bone deformation in children, it has grown to encompass a wide range of pathologic conditions, including age-induced wear and traumatic injuries. Treatment has progressed from the use of plaster of Paris to immobilize injured limbs, to the introduction of X-rays, and then MRI, for diagnosis, to the developing use of 3D-printed joints.

What changes might be on the horizon, and how might orthopedics be practiced at the turn of the next century? The possibilities are astounding to our twenty-first-century minds.

ORTHOPEDICS IN THE FUTURE

It is the year 2100, and preventive medicine is now at the forefront of all health care. The artificial toxins that contribute to premature aging and disease have been identified and systematically removed from societies around the globe. Similarly, healthy lifestyle interventions have become the norm, and preventable illnesses no longer run rampant in our communities.

Medical care has been streamlined. Gone are the days of inaccessible, fragmented medical records; long-delayed referral requests; and hit-or-miss treatments that are delivered over months and years rather than days or hours. Real-time individual medical records accompany each patient in the form of an omni-accessible medical tattoo, and providers no longer have to struggle to treat a patient whose medical history is murky at best. Accurate records help obviate unnecessary tests, curtailing the financial cost of medical care. Global and hyperlocal population health metrics are combined with predictive analytics to pinpoint the medical interventions that have the highest probability of success for each individual. Pharmacogenetic identifiers detail which interventions are most likely to succeed, based on the genetic susceptibilities of each patient. Traditional surgical approaches with their risks and complications are nearly unheard of, and nanobiomechanics has become the standard of care. Finally, the long sought-after ideal of patient-centered care is approaching reality. The future is here.

PATIENT PROFILES

The following patient profiles explore what early twenty-second-century orthopedic practice might be like:

Arne is a 76 YO, born in 2024, who has been living in a remote agricultural community. The inhabitants of this community are skeptical of novel medical technologies and will not use the advanced preventive technologies that would derail many of the musculoskeletal ramifications of normal human aging. Arne has struggled with severe spinal stenosis with slowly worsening debility stemming from nerve damage that has caused leg weakness and a loss of balance. Arne's mobility has declined during the last 2 years, and he is no longer able to meet the arduous demands of his farm. As a result, he is motivated to explore what medical options may be available—but not without significant reservations regarding modern medicine.

After a consultation with his orthopedic specialist, he selects an option most in keeping with his own moral compass: old-fashioned (well, not quite!) surgery. His severe L1-L2 spinal stenosis is treated first with decompression performed by nano-robotic excavators. Sophisticated AI-directed nanobot printers then create a bone-based cellular matrix that is customized in situ and adapted in real time to Arne's individual biomechanical needs. This will provide a biodegradable scaffolding on which his own bone remodeling can be layered further. Because years of bony compression caused severe nerve injury, stem cell–directed nerve regeneration therapy will combine with nanorobotic local delivery of specialized enzymes to promote an ideal microenvironment for regrowth. The results? Repair of nerve injury that in our present world would have been permanent. In addition, Arne is able to once again actively contribute to the community he holds so dear.

Mika is a 50 YO tennis star, born in 2050. She has excelled beyond what athletes of her age could have achieved in an earlier era. Her career has spanned 35 years already and includes more than 21 titles. By many accounts, she is still at her peak, with multiple achievements coming after her 40th birthday. Mika has enjoyed a long and successful career made possible by the numerous preventive and regenerative technologies that were developed in the late twenty-first century.

Despite these regular interventions, with repeated high-intensity physical activity, she suffered an acute severe radial meniscal tear of her left knee. Her orthopedic specialist has recommended 24-hour nanorobotic therapy in which specialized medical nanobots will trim the torn, devitalized meniscal tissue and produce a collagen-based scaffold. They will then layer induced pluripotent stem cells on the scaffolding in conjunction with a nutritive growth-stimulating composite material, thus catalyzing the regeneration of meniscal tissue. Within 72 hours, healthy meniscal tissue will have replaced the damaged material and the patient will be cleared to begin physical activity. Her successful athletic career, rather than being cut short, will continue to thrive into the future.

Cam is a 35 YO naturalist and tour guide. Cam, similar to most people who live in the modern medical era, has an AGE-LESS (A Goal-Engineered Life-Extending Smart Server) personal care assistant (PCA). This is an AI–directed medical consultant with a multifaceted approach to helping individuals maintain health, providing personalized medical guidance from infancy onward. The goal of AGE-LESS is to promote lifelong habits that will support the development of a healthy, well-functioning body. By actively monitoring users' progress and providing real-time feedback, this holistic system gives each person the support they need to stay healthy.

Cam's AGE-LESS PCA has developed a continuous health plan that considers the specifics of their genetics and cellular health, as well as their activity level. The result is an approach that combines preventive and regenerative care to include seeding Cam's gut with laboratory-generated microorganisms that will live in harmony with their biome and help to reduce systemic inflammation while aiding more rapid healing. Cam has been issued a low-level laser therapy (LLLT) bodysuit that will deliver laser therapy in the comfort of their own home. The PCA coordinates with Cam's wellness nano-net, which monitors the body's inflammation levels and nociceptor activity, to schedule and administer therapy sessions.

Similar to many of the treatments that have become standard by 2100, LLLT therapy has a low side-effect profile, is cost-effective, and can safely be administered in the patient's home. These preventive interventions have become so mainstream that the term "patient" is rarely used; Cam, similar to so many others, is just a person who uses tech to maintain their health. Years of use have shown that these baseline interventions effectively reduce (or at least delay) the need for more invasive and life-altering treatments. Joint replacement therapy, for example, is an intervention of last resort and used only in cases of severe traumatic injury.

Omi is a rambunctious 4 YO whose parents used prenatal gene therapy to prevent hereditary osteogenesis imperfecta (OI), also known as brittle bone disease. Ground-breaking advancements in quantum computing and the sophistication of human cell culture technology have enabled scientists to solve delivery hurdles that held gene therapy back in the early twenty-first century. As a result, Omi is thriving, enjoying an active lifestyle with no symptoms of this debilitating condition. Moreover, she will not be able to pass OI down to her descendants.

On a recent visit to her grandparents' microfarm, Omi fell while climbing a tree. An injury that would have been life threatening without modern gene therapy was merely an inconvenience. Omi was an ideal candidate for the new RegenPod technology, which is a suspended-animation pod that allows for superfast bone healing in a controlled environment. Patient compliance is still a challenge in 2100, especially in active children who will not stay still long enough for their bones to heal properly, so the RegenPod has become a popular treatment mechanism.

This human-size treatment chamber allows patients to achieve superior bone healing while reducing impacts to their quality of life. Instead of being in a cast for weeks, a patient can spend 2 to 3 days in comfortable suspended animation while their bones are healed in situ. By carefully calibrating the stasis chamber and infusing the patient with a custom mix of nanochemical agents, optimal healing is achieved in the shortest period possible. The resulting healed bone is consistently free from complications and posttreatment infections while outperforming natural bone. For these reasons, the RegenPod has also become a popular option for professional athletes, who need to return to form as soon as possible.

SUMMARY

The future of medicine, orthopedics in particular, is full of potential. With time, gene therapy may be able to prevent a multitude of diseases, not only congenital disorders such as OI but also age-related diseases. Similarly, the medical application of nanotechnology has barely begun but it too is alluring in its promise to help fight disease and promote health. What other technologies are yet unimagined but beckon to us from the future? As medical researchers and frontline practitioners both focus on delivering more advanced and more effective treatments, maintaining a focus on accessibility, patient-centered care, and cost-effectiveness will ensure that the greatest number of people can benefit. In that way, the promise of a healthier future can be shared by all.

DISCLOSURE

Disclosure of any relationship with a commercial company that has a direct financial interest in subject matter or materials discussed in article or with a company making a competing product: None.

FURTHER READING

Jordan S. Interventional Orthopedics: The future of musculoskeletal injury treatment. DigitalCommons@SHU. https://digitalcommons.sacredheart.edu/acadfest/2022/all/142/.

Beaty JH. The future of orthopedics. Journal of Orthopaedic Science 2009;14(3):245–7.

Bini SA, Schilling PL, Patel S, et al. Digital Orthopaedics: A glimpse into the future in the midst of a pandemic. Journal of Arthroplasty 2020;35(7):S68–73.

Hines L. What innovations could shape the future of orthopaedics? - Orthopaedic Product News. Orthopaedic Product News 2021. Available at: https://www.opnews.com/2021/06/what-innovations-could-shape-the-future-of-orthopaedics/17025.

Rojas Y. Future trends in the field of orthopedics | Orthopaedic Associates of Central Maryland. Orthopaedic Associates of Central Maryland 2022. Available at: https://www.mdbonedocs.com/future-trends-in-the-field-of-orthopedics/.

Orthopedics. Available at: https://lancastermedicalheritagemuseum.org/wp-content/themes/edward-hand/vm/vex18/index.htm.

Szostakowski B, Smitham P, Khan W. Plaster of Paris–Short history of casting and injured limb immobilzation. The Open Orthopaedics Journal 2017;11(1):291–6.

Szostakowski B, Smitham P, Khan W. Plaster of Paris–Short history of casting and injured limb immobilzation. The Open Orthopaedics Journal 2017;11(1):291–6.

Arthritis Society. 3D printing for joint regeneration (Bioprinting). Arthritis Society. Available at: https://arthritis.ca/treatment/emerging-treatment-and-research/3d-printing-to-regenerate-joints#:~:text=However%2C%20in%20a%20new%20method, successive%20micro%2Dlayers%20of%20materials.

Moving?

Make sure your subscription moves with you!

To notify us of your new address, find your **Clinics Account Number** (located on your mailing label above your name), and contact customer service at:

Email: journalscustomerservice-usa@elsevier.com

800-654-2452 (subscribers in the U.S. & Canada)
314-447-8871 (subscribers outside of the U.S. & Canada)

Fax number: 314-447-8029

Elsevier Health Sciences Division
Subscription Customer Service
3251 Riverport Lane
Maryland Heights, MO 63043

*To ensure uninterrupted delivery of your subscription, please notify us at least 4 weeks in advance of move.

Printed and bound by CPI Group (UK) Ltd, Croydon, CR0 4YY

03/10/2024

01040466-0015